PHILOSOPHY OF HATHA YOGA

Second Edition, Revised and Expanded

D0881987

PHILOSOPHY OF HATHA YOGA

Second Edition, Revised and Expanded

Pandit Usharbudh Arya,D.Litt.

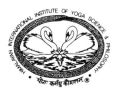

The Himalayan International Institute
of Yoga Science and Philosophy of the U.S.A.
Honesdale, Pennsylvania

Second Edition, Revised and Expanded
First printing June 1985

Copyright 1977, 1985 by
The Himalayan International Institute
of Yoga Science and Philosophy of the U.S.A.
RR 1, Box 400
Honesdale, Pennsylvania 18431

ISBN 0-89389-088-X
Printed in the United States of America.

Library of Congress Cataloging in Publication Data

Arya, Usharbudh.
    Philosophy of hatha yoga.

    1. Yoga, Hatha. I. Title.
RA781.7.A78   1984   613.7'046   84-19790

Contents

OM
Gurubhyo namah
Parampara-gurubhyo namah
Parameshthi-gurave namah

Homage to my Gurus—
    the first Guru, my mother
    the second Guru, my father
    the third Gurus, all my teachers
    —from a fly to all writers
    whose books I have read

Homage to the Gurus of my lineage—
    through H. H. Swami Rama

Homage to the Supreme Absolute Guru.

OM

Preface

The yoga science is one. Just as various specialties in one medical science do not separate medical sciences, so the various specialties within yoga do not make many yogas. Hatha yoga, laya yoga, nada yoga, mantra yoga, kundalini yoga, and so forth are simply various emphases to help perfect different areas of human personality, in different stages of an aspirant's development. All these should be seen within the single framework of raja yoga, which is the yoga of eight complements, as promulgated by Patanjali. Of these, hatha yoga has become the most popular and practically synonymous with the totality of yoga. The reason for this is that most human beings identify the self with the physical body, and for this reason the majority have to begin their journey to the spiritual self in the vehicle called the body. To make the vehicle the goal of the journey is obviously erroneous. The vehicle is run through the infusion and interaction of subtler forces and essences. The practice of hatha yoga is incomplete unless some of these subtler forces and essences such as mind and prana are understood. The moment these forces are understood, the practice of hatha yoga unblocks the channels through which these essences are infused into the body during the practice of hatha. Without this, hatha merely becomes another system of physical exercise.

For those teaching within the lineage of succession from and the tradition of the Himalayan masters—the only living authorities on yoga—it is imperative that yoga should not be reduced merely to another set of physical exercises. The science of yoga should remain a method for gaining the higher ground of awareness. It must also be understood that without this awareness of subtler essences the exercise itself will be incomplete and the practitioner will gain neither the sole mastery nor full benefits from its practice.

The most authentic text of hatha yoga—like Patanjali's work is for raja yoga—is *Hatha-yoga-pradipika* of Svatmarama. Like all other Sanskrit texts of hatha yoga, *Hatha-yoga-pradipika* emphatically supports our view. We read the following statements of Svatmarama:

> This science of hatha yoga shines brilliant and serves like a ladder for a seeker aspiring to climb to the highest in raja yoga. (I.1)

> The science of hatha is taught only for the sake of raja yoga. (I.2)

> All the practices of hatha should be observed only till their fruit, raja yoga, is gained. (I.67)

> Hatha without raja yoga and raja yoga without hatha cannot be accomplished, therefore one should practice them together until perfection is reached. (II. 76)

> Those who practice only hatha and do not know raja yoga—I consider such practitioners to be depriving themselves of the fruit of their endeavor. (IV.79)

All the systems of hatha yoga and laya yoga help the
achievement of raja yoga. He who has climbed to raja
yoga can deceive time and master death. (IV.103)

A careful reader of the texts of hatha yoga including the
one by Svatmarama cannot fail to be impressed by the
references to the role the mind plays in hatha yoga and yet
it is strange that nowadays much of hatha is taught without
the mental exercises that alone can make the body of a
hatha yogi vibrant as does an electric current the copper
wire. Just as Svatmarama's work begins with the statement
quoted above that the purpose of hatha yoga is to lead to
the heights of raja yoga, it ends as follows:

> Until the prana enters the middle path [of the *sushumna*
>   stream],
> Until the point [of concentration] becomes firm through
>   the control of prana,
> Until one's essence flows naturally and evenly in
>   meditation,
> Till then all your knowledge [of hatha] is myth,
>   hypocrisy, and words.

In my study of the Sanskrit texts of hatha yoga, I was
puzzled as to why the masters composing these texts were
using what is known in grammar as the optative mood in
the construction of their verb forms, which can be
translated both as "one should do it this way" or "one
habitually does so." It was only through the grace of
Gurudev that the puzzle was solved. The science of hatha
yoga first appeared as records of physical experiences that
occurred naturally when mind and prana have entered the
sushumna stream of the kundalini in the practice of
meditation. The yogi's body does habitually and naturally
what a beginner in hatha yoga is advised to do by way of an

endeavor. It is from this experience that our hatha-kundalini sutras in chapter 6 of the present volume first came forth. The first five chapters may be read both as an introduction to and as a commentary on these sutras. It is hoped that by this effort even the easiest practices of hatha yoga will be elevated to an inner spiritual experience and the subtler essences of the practitioner's personality will suffuse the body of the practitioner with immortal energy, that is, *amrita*.

I am most grateful to Michael Smith of the Center for Higher Consciousness, Minneapolis, Minnesota, for editing this volume and to Lalita Devi, my wife, for further refining the work. My gratitude flows to the staff of the Himalayan Institute, whose anonymous service makes the Gurudev's work possible.

In this work all that is beneficial proceeds from the Guru lineage and all that is erroneous is mine.

USHARBUDH ARYA

1

Watching the Mind
Watching the Body

Most people practice hatha yoga not for its philosophy but for its physical benefits. Their attention is limited to the outer container rather than the inner content of personality. In actual history, however, the hatha exercises were developed within the framework of *Ashtanga* yoga, the Yoga of the Eight Limbs, and were meant to train the disciple for higher, deeper, spiritual disciplines.

The human personality exists and functions on manifold levels, and because of this, the word *hatha,* like many other Sanskrit words relating to the study of the personality, has multiple meanings. In any philosophical study in the Sanskrit language, we can take a meaning that applies on one level of our understanding, grasp that meaning, master that ground, and then leave it behind. If we rise further, the same word on a second level will convey an entirely different meaning. So the meaning of the word changes as we progress from ground to ground.

The grossest meaning of the word *hatha* is force, forcing, doing something forcibly, because initially hatha is almost forcing ourselves to break a body habit. If, for example, the body has the habit of slouching, forcing that

1

habit out and forcing a new habit in is hatha. But it is a gentle forcing. It is not the forcing like that of a wrestler or a weightlifter. So, when one begins to understand from where that gentle part of the forcing comes, the meaning of *hatha* shifts and then one is thinking not of the physical body alone but of subtler truths, cosmic truths, the universal energy fields, the sun and the moon. The word *ha* means the sun; the word *tha* means the moon. As the understanding of one's personal, physical relationship with the universe begins to dawn, again the meaning shifts, and the sun is not the sun that rises at six o'clock in the morning, and the moon is not the moon that shines in the sky at night. The sun is the active, "masculine," right nostril breath and the moon is the intuitive, "feminine," left nostril breath. In this way one finds that the practice of hatha yoga is working simultaneously on various levels.

The people, thousands upon thousands of years ago, who developed the science, philosophy, and practice of hatha yoga were masters of what, in the Buddhist philosophy, is called one of the *paramitas,* the ten perfections required of a Buddha or enlightened spiritual being. One of those ten is *kaushala* or expertise in the means of liberating others. They had one principle always in mind. It was what my father, when he was teaching me as a child, always said: "If you have fallen in mud, you cannot lie there and say, 'I wish I could rise instead from the floor of the Taj Mahal.' " If you have fallen in mud, you have to put your hands down again in mud and get up from the mud. Having fallen in mud, you cannot rise from a marble floor.

So, at present human beings have their consciousness fixed at various levels of reality. Whatever they identify with in their life, whatever is their conception of Self, from that point they must begin. In dealing with all their problems, they must start from that point. That is what is real and important to them. There are many people to whom the idea of achieving the perfection of an enlightened being and so on is just vague mystifying speech devised by those strange, inscrutable Easterners who come over here and confuse us. So what a teacher of yoga does is start exactly with whatever it is that a person identifies with. If someone is interested in machines, he may use biofeedback yoga. If someone else begins with a problem of chemical dependency, he may start with developing will power; if someone else wants to maintain a youthful appearance, then he may start with hatha postures and diet; and so on.

In yoga philosophy there are five sheaths around the spiritual self of man—the outermost first sheath is known as *annamaya,* made up of the food that we eat. The second sheath is the finer essence of the food, the *pranamaya* sheath made of the vital force. The third sheath is the *manomaya,* a further essence of prana, the mental essence. The *vijnanamaya,* the fourth sheath, is made of limited consciousness. And the fifth sheath is the *anandamaya,* the sheath made of limited pleasure (limitations placed on joy).

The average individual is more conscious of his outermost sheath, the *annamaya kosha,* the food sheath or physical body. We speak of ourselves and we put our hand on our chest! We say, "I am hungry." We are not speaking of the mind's hunger but of the hunger of the body. So there is this physical identification. Where does control of this physical body fit in the entire philosophy of yoga? Its purpose is to gradually draw the attention from the grosser parts of us to the finer ones. Ordinarily we use our body and are not even conscious that the body is being used. In any crowded room people are in so many different postures, yet only a few may be aware of their postures. Unless it is mentioned, it does not occur to people to look at themselves and say, "Ah, I'm sitting in this posture." The primary consideration, therefore, in the practice of hatha yoga philosophically is the practice of mindfulness, self-observation, the habit of being a witness to one's own physical functions, aware of whatever it is that we are doing with our bodies, whether it be the external surfaces of the body or internal things like muscle tension, heart rate, bloodflow, and breathing. A lot of people identify with their appearance, and they have some "beauty in a bottle" lotion which they apply to their face. They are keenly aware of the external surface of the body, but they are not at all conscious of their postures. People seldom say to themselves, "Here I am lying down; here I am sitting up; here I am standing; here I am walking, now I am lifting my foot, now I am putting it down. This is what is happening to the base of the spine as I am moving my foot from one spot to the next, as I am walking, or shuffling at a bus stop." This mindfulness in daily life is something that is a starting point in the philosophy of *sakshi*, the philosophy of being a witness, of being aware of the body from head to toe. Now, at this moment, are you aware of everything in you? What is the position of the scalp? What sensations do you have there at this moment? Exactly what is the position of the muscles of the forehead? In this way, if you are really a witness to your body, you are mastering deeper hatha.

But the body is just the external surface. As a yogi advances in the practice of mindfulness, his state of being a witness grows further, even to so-called "unconscious" functions. People today have become much more aware of autonomic functions, but to a great yogi there is no such thing as an autonomic function. There is no such thing as automatic heartbeats. Instead he says, "I can reduce it or I can increase it." He progressively becomes aware not only of the external, physical skeleton but also of all the internal organs. As a yogi advances through the practice of hatha yoga he becomes aware of his internal organs. He knows the condition of his lungs, and if there is any kind of disease there, he recognizes it.

Sometimes subtle information such as this comes to us symbolically. We gain access to this information involuntarily and accidentally in dreams, but we do not understand it. The relationship of body and mind in one respect is forgotten during the dreams, but in another respect it is even more emphasized. This is so because in the dream the mind is not at a standstill, but is moving around within the confines of the personality without any input from the outside through the senses. All that the mind can do, if the dream has any kind of rationality to it, is to examine that part of the mind which is in the body. Quite often in the dream, a superior part of the mind examines a lower part of the mind which is permeating the body. For instance, sometimes one may dream of crossing a river or of floating down a river. What is actually happening is that the mind is inspecting the river of a certain artery or vein and comes to a junction where another river is meeting it. The dreamer may even come to a waterfall or rapids and feel that he is getting dumped somewhere; he may taste the saltiness of the blood itself. Or he may find an obstacle such as a fallen tree, but instead of that being an ordinary tree outside that you had seen or were afraid of, it turns out to be in reality a blood clot.

Every gross object and the experience of anything

gross in the world is a pointer to something finer and less visible. Every shape, every form, every hexagon and triangle, every object, everything that is experienced with the physical body, points to something finer within. And because our language is tied down to only visible things, and because the abstract things do not so readily impress themselves upon our minds, our language is full of gross ideas, concrete things. Abstract things do come to the mind when they are expressed in the language of symbols. The gross thing we see points to the subtle unseen thing. A tree across a river is much more real to us than a clot in an artery. What we see in a dream then is not a clot in an artery but the symbol, a slight shift, a transference of meaning, a transference of form from something less visible to something more visible, something more concrete that the mind will readily recognize. Therefore it sees not the clot in the artery but a log or a rock blocking the stream.

Unless you understand the functioning of the mind, you cannot understand the functioning of the body at all. The reading of a textbook on physiology or anatomy is not understanding the body. If it were so, eighty percent to one hundred percent of our diseases would not be psychosomatic. So to understand the philosophy of hatha yoga one first needs to deal with the mind: its state, its attitude, its mood.

As a yogi refines himself he becomes more conscious of all the functions of his body—what is happening in the stomach, the liver, the kidneys. One of the reasons the yogis devised the methods of internal cleansing was that when they sat down to meditate, even the slightest particle in the ducts or in the intestines was felt to be present and caused the mind to become distracted. That irritant had to be removed. Hatha yoga, therefore, was devised by raja yogis as a process of both physiological and psychological purification for the practice of meditation. Such things as sweating or cleansing of the lymph nodes and other glands, exhaling of all carbon dioxide, and all the washes are also purifications preparatory to meditation.

The yogis who wrote about the philosophy of hatha yoga said that as they tried to purify their bodies they became more aware of the utter hopelessness of really making them good, clean, and beautiful. They said, "We have looked over and over this body and have applied all kinds of purification processes, and we can find nothing beautiful in it. Through our constant efforts of purification we have become more and more aware of all the ugliness that we store in it." One of the contemplations in the Buddhist meditation system is *ahare patikula-sanna* in the Pali language. In Sanskrit, it is known as *ahare pratikula-sanjna,* a distaste for food because of awareness of the digestive processes involved. The purificatory processes of internal washes not only cleanse the body inside to keep it healthy but also remind one of the constant necessity of doing it. For example, each time one overeats, one is made aware of the extra work and effort it will take to once again purify the body.

I myself come from a part of India which is known for its delicious foods. The people there are known for their hospitality in terms of food. I have always enjoyed good food, but in the last year or so I have become so aware of the adverse effects of eating on the mind that I have reached a point where I cannot with a clear conscience eat more than small amounts at a time. The moment I take my food, I notice a shift occurring. My breath becomes heavier, and the finer kundalini currents become gross, and it takes at least two or three hours of great mental concentration to sit down and meditate or conduct a meditation for others. I have to again purify my mind. And by purifying my mind, I mean refining the finer currents of the mental energy that flow through the body. The intake of food immediately makes it *tamasic,* makes it gross. This is not to say that you should not eat. As one progresses in yoga, some things will naturally develop. Sensitivity to food is one of them. Hatha yoga is a process of developing that sensitivity to the external surfaces of the body as well as to the internal organs of the body and all the inner functions.

You understand hatha yoga if you understand it as a preparation for spiritual liberation. In this volume different aspects of hatha will be analyzed to see where they fit in the higher philosophy and how they lead to higher consciousness. Higher consciousness does not merely mean an immediate awareness of the extent of this great ever-going universe, the *jagat.* It also means an immediate awareness of godliness. There is a passage: *Shariram-adyam khalu dharma-sadhanam,* "The body indeed is the primary tool for gaining virtue." The body is weak and yet there is a desire to achieve great things. How can that be done? If, as the ancient texts say, the body is the first means of the practice of virtue and righteousness, then the body should be preserved. There is no other reason for this body to be preserved. There is no other beauty in it. If you scratch the surface of your skin, what beauty do you find in there?

From the grosser to the finer, there is the body, the internal organs, the breath, the prana or vital force, the mind that is in the body, the mind that remembers the body and physical events, and finally the higher mind. The progress in the practice of hatha is from the external levels gradually to the internal levels. What does that mean? It means first of all, become more and more conscious of the different levels and slowly shift the mind's identification from one level to a finer one. Therefore, you progressively remove the control that the grosser has over the finer parts of your being and establish control of the finer over the relatively grosser parts of your being.

Let us take, for example, the most material and lowest part of our being, the external surfaces of the body that we consider to be beautiful. The position of our physical body affects something finer, and that is the internal system. If someone sits slouching, he immediately inhibits the internal organs. He also inhibits the finer functions such as the breath and spiritual functions such as the free flow of the kundalini force. Or if someone uses a poor position when having a bowel movement, he inhibits the natural functions of those organs.

India has many unhygienic habits but there are some that are comparatively more hygienic than some habits in the West. It is a common custom in the West for men to stand to urinate. In India this is regarded as a sign of Western laziness. Indians squat on two feet in the same position in which they sit for the bowel movement. The Western system of toilet stools is not known, except recently in the modern cities. Indians feel standing is a poor position because it does not fully empty the kidneys; it does not put the right pressure against the body to accomplish complete evacuation. The same is true for the Western position of sitting for the bowel movement. It is a very unnatural position and leads to all kinds of problems such as constipation and hemorrhoids.

We see, then, how just the positioning of the external

physical body affects our internal organs. Anybody knows this, but it is a question of becoming aware of it and of living one's life day to day in terms of this knowledge. Stopping that inhibition that is placed by the external on the internal, by the gross on the finer, is part of being aware. As soon as you identify not merely with the surfaces of the body, not merely with the comfort of the skeleton, your philosophy changes. Observe the chairs found in cars and airplanes. It is such a torture to travel. I have a busy life so I use cars and planes for my time for meditation. I have not yet found a car in which I can sit down and really feel comfortable and straight to meditate. I just do not know how to put my spine in the right place to use my hours in the airplane for meditation because the seat has been designed by people who are only aware of the comfort of the external skeleton or the muscles and this strange kind of shape that the body takes with people who have not trained their bodies. When you are aware of the internal organs and what is happening to them at any given moment you can't sit in a car comfortably and you can't sit on a couch or a sofa comfortably and you cannot sleep on a soft bed comfortably. So your whole concept of the benefits of modern civilization changes.

The awareness of the needs of the internal organs will then determine the positioning of the external physical body. This is especially so for finer functions, such as the breath. Few pieces of furniture at all in modern civilization are designed to help people remember breath. No good breath habit is formed. Later one's identification has to change again; an awareness of prana and then the awareness of the mind as functioning in the physical body must develop. Remember the example of the dream state.

Some of this deeper awareness can be felt in the

relaxation exercises that are done in the corpse posture, which enhances one's awareness of the mind in the body: relax the mind that is in the forehead, and the muscle of your forehead relaxes; relax the mind that is in the cheeks, and your cheeks relax; relax the portion of your mind that is in your shoulders, and your shoulders relax. Gradually one moves from the grosser to the finer.

Yoga is unlike any other system of exercise. The movements are done slowly. There is constant self-observation; if we do not have constant self-observation, then obviously we are not doing the hatha properly. It is not absolutely necessary to have only slow movements, but to have full observation in fast movements too. For example, if you have proper concentration, you can keep your eyes fixed on your fingertip as you move it quickly to and fro. If you ever have the chance to watch an Indian dancer, watch the eyes. Some of the exercises given to the dancers preparing them in childhood—they start training them at the age of three—are very similar to the self-observation practices of hatha yoga.

The muscles, the skeleton, the nerves, the breath, and the mind are all coordinated and function together at the same time. Unless a student of hatha bears those five things in mind during a given exercise, he will not be able to do the exercise correctly.

When you are practicing a hatha yoga position, practice it first in your mind:

> Close your eyes. Relax your mind and your forehead and visualize yourself lying down. Just see yourself lying down, and imagine yourself in that position bringing your feet together with your hands resting by your sides.

Turn the palms over, placing the back of the hands on the ground.

Slowly lift your feet without bending your knees. Bend from the hips and gradually lift the legs to a position perpendicular to the floor. Breathe slowly while in that position.

Now, keeping the position, without bending your knees, observe what effect it has on your abdominal muscles. Observe what effect it is having on the navel and stomach area.

Continue to observe your breathing in that position. Continue to observe the effect on all the muscles and again without bending your knees, slowly lower your feet and gently place them on the ground.

Relax your body. Feel the breath flowing through your entire body from head to toe while you are still lying on the ground. Open your eyes.

This was just a simple leg lift leading to the shoulderstand posture, but it doesn't matter what the position is; you can do it over and over and you can see the effect on the mind. The more you relax, the easier your visualization is; you can perfect a posture without ever moving your body! The lazy man's guide to hatha yoga! An excellent course in hatha yoga without any visual aid can be done in this way, provided we have right words and describe the right angles and do it in the mind.

From your standpoint it would seem as if we were thinking of the body and then transferring that thought to the mind in a mental state. But actually, where the functioning of human consciousness is concerned, consciousness comes first, the body comes second. Is it not so? If you had no consciousness what would you be? A corpse. So it is the mind that trains the body. What is done ordinarily in hatha yoga classes is training the mind by first training the body. When a person actually places his body in a certain position, what he is doing is making the mind experience that position. This is a roundabout way of training the mind; it is only for the non-meditative people whose identification is primarily with the physical shape rather than the mental function.

If one's identification is with the physical shape, he should start with the physical shape. Naturally the mind that is in the body experiences that shape in thought. If we place our arm in a particular situation, we are doing two things. One, we are giving it that shape and, two, we are having our mind experience that geometrical formation. We are impressing upon our mind that geometrical formation and are creating a *mandala* or a *yantra*. The whole art and science of mandalas is making the mind experience a geometrical form.

The question might be asked whether the exercises done purely mentally would give the same benefits as doing them physically, and the answer is that in the long run it could, but there are some very basic physiological benefits that cannot wait. If, however, one spent ten minutes every day doing nothing but contemplating an erect spine, one would form the habit of an erect spine. Whenever a student has difficulty mastering a posture, for example, it is well to have him go over the posture in the mind, over and over.

Hatha yoga then builds a bridge from the body to the deepest recesses of the mind which deal with geometry, with form, with memory, and which send forth the commands to control the entire autonomic system. That is only one step.

The use of the mind in doing the physical exercises can be seen as follows:

Close your eyes and completely relax your skull muscles and forehead muscles.

Relax your eyebrows, eyes; relax your cheeks, relax your jaw.

Relax your neck, shoulders; relax your shoulders until you feel the relaxation in your fingertips.

Relax your cardiac center; relax your shoulders; relax your neck; relax your jaw; relax your cheeks; relax your forehead.

Without removing your relaxation of the forehead, imagine the forehead muscles and scalp muscles being lifted up. Keep the forehead relaxed; just in your mind lift the scalp and forehead muscles. You'll find you will immediately become conscious of any tension rising in the forehead.

Relax your whole face and breathe slowly and smoothly.

Feeling your breath, imagine that you are turning your neck slowly to the left while inhaling. Bring your neck as far to the left as you comfortably can and feel all the tension that arises in the neck muscles.

Exhaling slowly, bring your neck back to the center. Keep your neck muscles relaxed physically.

Now inhaling, move your neck mentally to the right. Slowly move it to the right along with the breath, feeling the breath in the nostrils, feeling all the tensions in the muscles, but physically keeping the neck relaxed. Bring it as far to the right as you comfortably can, as if trying to look over your right shoulder. Feel the tension to the point of the threshold of pain.

Then relax those muscles and slowly exhale, and feeling the breath in the nostrils, bring the neck back to the center. Inhale and exhale slowly and smoothly, and open your eyes.

When you have done that mentally, then do it physically. Observe what the mind is doing; how it is observing the finest muscles and tissues. Observe the mind commanding the muscles to move slowly.

Remain aware of the breath and how the mind is aware of the breath. Let the higher mind observe the part of the mind that is aware of the breath. Know that "I am aware of the breath" and that "I am aware of the tension that is taking place in the muscles."

Try to see which of the finer muscles and tissues that you are not normally aware of, you now become aware of, and try to isolate them in your mind. Let it be a lesson in self-anatomy.

Just continue to observe how the mind is using this awareness of the breath. Observe how the mind is sending the impulses and orders into those muscles.

Let it be an exercise in thinking, not in doing. How is the mind thinking this movement? Observe the movement. See every movement as from one point to the immediately adjacent point. Observe each point in that circular movement. Fill in the mental part as you are doing it.

Move your hand at random.
Now watch the movement with your eyes.
Now close your eyes and watch the movement.
Does the movement make sense?

Make any movement for the length of an exhalation, one movement for the length of an exhalation, and watch your mind moving. Observe how the mind observes the movement along with the breath.

At each level of the practice, there is something of the mind, something of the body, something of the kundalini—it depends on what you do with your mind. For example, most people try to do their asanas and even the joints and glands exercises by moving their bodies alone. This is even true of some teachers. The principle we have repeatedly emphasized is that the movement of the body is at birth it's the opposite!

nothing, and that movement of the mind is everything. The mind governs the movement of the body. It is the mind that moves; then the body follows. You watch that movement of the body which is from the movement of the mind. So every physical exercise is, first, a mental exercise. This applies to the simple joints and glands exercises as well as to the asanas. Here is an example of the kind of awareness to cultivate during your actual practice:

> Close your eyes and relax your forehead. Relax your facial muscles. Relax the shoulders.
> Send the order only to the point where movement is felt all the way down in the fingertips. The fingers are ready to rise but do not rise. Observe! Now relax all the way from the shoulders to the fingertips.
> Keep your eyes closed. Send an order to the arm to move. Feel the order going down. Feel tension building from the shoulders to the fingertips. Let your hand rise just ever so slightly, just to reduce the pressure on your leg where your hand was resting. Put the hand back again and relax. Relax all the way from the brain to the fingertips.
> Now observe the order to move going down from the brain to the shoulders, to the fingertips, and lift your hand ever so slightly. Lift it up. Watch it moving. Very slowly straighten your hand; watch it straightening. Feel every tissue in the hand. Now feel every tissue relaxing slowly and the hand going down, back again. Let all the muscles relax again.
> Open your eyes.

We did not do even one complete joints and glands exercise, but you could see what can be learned by observing the movement. If you had observed the complete movement, what would you have felt? Some people who are teaching joints and glands exercises have not quite mastered this habit of self-observation. If I do joints and glands exercises, I watch each movement, each point of the movement, from one point to the next point—what is happening to my finger, what is happening to every minute muscle in the hand, how the hand is straightening, how the arm is straightening, how the elbows are straightening, what I feel in each muscle, each minute area. This way I learn something about my anatomy. Then if, for instance, I have a headache, I can know what part of my anatomy it affects.

When you are practicing hatha, do it as a thought process. The body will much more easily obey you. Whenever you are practicing hatha, whether you are the teacher or the student, accomplish it first in your mind as a thought process.

> Close your eyes. Sit straight. Think of yourself bending forward without curving the spine, as if it were moving from the pelvis, until you are well forward.
>
> Slowly go down. In your mind, see yourself bending forward from the hips and touching the shin area below the knees with your nose.
>
> Remain in this position for a few breaths and then slowly sit up. Straighten slowly, breathing in until your spine is completely straight.
>
> Again, exhale. Bend forward in your mind and gradually, slowly, touch the nose to the shin and observe what is happening in your stomach area; what is happening to your spine as you are in that posture.
>
> Mentally cross your hands behind your back and just observe yourself in that position; what is happening with each muscle?
>
> Rise up, inhaling slowly. As you rise up, feel what is happening with your thighs, your stomach muscles, your sides, your lungs, and what is happening with your breathing.

Relax your shoulders and arms completely, and without allowing any tension in your shoulder, mentally lift your right arm so that the back of your head is under the chin. Keep your arm relaxed.
Slowly stretch your arm out forward and watch yourself doing so.
Open your eyes.

With all of these exercises it is the movement of the mind that initiates physical movement. It is with a thought that a movement begins, and it is then that your anatomy moves—even before the first flicker of tension is felt in the shoulder blades. When the signal goes out from the mind to move the arm, in what tissues does the first flicker occur after the signal has left the brain? Do not move the muscle. Observe the movement of the mind; in your mind you move it. You do this all the time without realizing it because it happens so quickly that you do not dwell on it.

Relax your shoulders and all the rest of you. Without letting the slightest tension build in the shoulders, observe the mind sending forth only the order to move the arm. Stop immediately as soon as you begin to feel the first tension that is the beginning of the movement of the body. Observe the order going down; then stop the order, countermand the order. Keep your shoulders and the neck completely relaxed. Your mind sends the order to move; you watch the order go and yet you do not move. Do not allow the slightest tension to build there. (Unless you have mastered your relaxation exercises, you will have difficulty with doing this.)
Now obey the order only to the extent of the slightest tension arising which begins a movement. When you do it physically, you will have better mastery of it.

Again, close your eyes. Relax your face.

Relax your forehead; relax your face; relax your jaw.

Relax your shoulders. Relax your cardiac center.

Breathe slowly and easily and think of yourself standing with feet slightly apart. Think of yourself joining your hands in front of your cardiac center and pressing the cardiac center with the bony ridges of your thumbs.

Watch your breath. Be aware of the position of your spine as you are standing. Raise up your arms so that your ears are between your arms.

Stretch up and look up to the sun. All the beautiful energy of the whole universe is flowing into you, for the energy and light in you is the same as the light in the sun, and you think: I am the sun. Slowly move forward and bend not from the middle of the spine but from the hips. Bend forward farther and farther and see yourself touching your forehead to your shins, your hands to the sides of your feet on the ground.

Maintain that position and observe what is happening to your spine, what is happening with your breath, where the exertions and tensions in your shoulders and knees are.

Slowly rise up again and straighten up from the waist.

Open your eyes.

Master it as a thought process and then you will know exactly what you are supposed to do with the body. You would not even need a teacher. The movement of the body is nothing. It is only the movement of the mind.

With every movement you make in the course of the day—everywhere—if you can be aware of the movement, you will walk as if twenty-four hours you were dancing. That is how classical Indian dancing developed out of temple worship rituals. The people were taught to move with the awareness. For example, the sipping of sacred water is a preparation for any temple ritual. Water is filled in the palm and taken; and it is taken again. All the while one is observing the body and observing where the water is going. The water is taken with the left hand and touched to various limbs with fingers of the right hand. One is observing the movement, observing the limbs, observing the senses and how the senses experience the touch of water and how the movement is going from point to point, how each point of the body is touched. And that ritual itself becomes a dance. Any act, any movement of the body, is a dance. That becomes so not by attending a dance school, but by watching the mind watching the body.

2

Worship

We shall discuss here three approaches to hatha yoga: *tapas* (ascetic practice), worship, and the evolution of mind.

There is a word *kriya* yoga, which means "yoga of practice." Kriya yoga is any course in yoga, a complete course in which there is a little mental practice. It may be practice of mantra, of meditation, of speech, of asanas, or of certain moral standards. In the Yoga Sutras, which is the major text of yoga, the first sutra, the first aphorism, the first sentence, of the second chapter defines kriya yoga. And in defining kriya yoga, the first component of the definition is tapas.

The word *tapas* means ascetic practice, a concentrated practice, to go toward something with utmost concentration. To undertake something with a little bit of sweat and effort is tapas. The word *tapas* actually comes from heat or heating up, and any practice should have a little of tapas in it. The word *hatha* is not used by the ancient author, master, Patanjali of the Yoga Sutras. He uses the word *tapas,* heating oneself up, sweating a little with intense concentration, putting as much of oneself into it as possible.

The word *tapas* also occurs as one of the five *niyamas.* In the practice of raja yoga, the second rung among the eight rungs is *niyama.* Now, of the five *niyamas* or principles/rules of behavior, the third one is *tapas.* Asceticism. Asceticism does not always mean sleeping on the bare ground or going without food in the desert. Rather, it simply means exertion of your total personality, intense concentration with a definite goal, with a certain something in front of you and pushing yourself just a little—one step more than you did yesterday. Without tapas there is no purification.

As anyone practicing hatha yoga has experienced, doing the asanas requires intense concentration so that one is aware of every minor, fine tissue of the part of the body that is being exercised. But the purpose and goal of tapas is to attain an intense one-pointed state of mind. When you exert yourself and repeatedly do something, whether you do it physically as in the case of hatha or you do it with the mouth as in the case of chanting or uttering of a mantra or repeating something to memorize it, or whether you do it only mentally, ultimately your mind becomes fixed on it. Until the mind is fixed on something, until that something has gone into the depths of your subconscious, that act, whatever it is, remains artificial. It remains separate from the body, separate from life. It is something that is being artificially induced and is not natural, like a student driver who is very conscious of shifting the gear, holding the steering wheel, pushing the brakes, pushing the accelerator, removing the foot, watching here, looking there— there are just so many things to do. Very confusing. But by doing it over and over and over again, what happens? You are hardly conscious of what you are doing when driving. Or, for example, you have moved, and the first time you have to remember the street; second time, you still have to remember the street; third or fourth time, you leave your office in the afternoon and you end up in front of your previous house. Just force of habit made you turn there. But after a while it becomes natural to arrive at the new home.

So tapas is that attitude in life through which, by doing something repeatedly and exerting oneself repeatedly, one makes something a definite part of one's inner mind. Sometimes an act of tapas may be undertaken just to strengthen the mind by doing something that is slightly unpleasant and learning to conquer the distinctions our minds have between pain and pleasure.

For example, there is the case of a practicing yogi who took the vow that he would stand for twelve years. He did not sit or lie down for twelve years. I think his disciples forced him to make a compromise. They made a platform, a board, that he could only lean on. Now, what is the purpose of an act like that? It is in the same category as your waking up at 6 a.m. tomorrow morning and 6 a.m. day after tomorrow morning and for four days and for four months and for four years and for forty years, and discovering that your mind has the strength to do such things. By doing it over and over, you realize the existence of that strength in your mind.

After two or three years of doing it, it is no longer an exertion. It has now become a purification. The mind no longer has the sloth, no longer has the negligent attitude. By doing it over and over, through a little force (*ha-tha*), by pushing yourself just a little, you change the habit of your mind, and where the mind sometimes would sleep until 10 a.m., sometimes until 8 a.m., now after extended repetition you have broken the habit of the mind. Now 6 a.m. is

purification — when you condition
yourself for, or beyond, t
overcome a short coming or weakness

24   *Philosophy of Hatha Yoga*

normal and natural, and a certain purification of the mind
has been attained; a certain undesirable quality that was in
the mind has been cast off. Then when you have reached
that point of purification, when you have conquered that
part of slothfulness, that impurity, you say, "Now where
do I go next?" And you set yourself another little goal, such
as conquest of the body.

Hatha yoga is conquest of the body. Everyone goes out
conquering the rest of the world. The greatest conquest in
the world is self-conquest, and for an average person that
begins with conquest of the body. There are very few
people who first conquer the mind and thereby conquer
the body; as I said earlier, they have to start from the
ground where they have fallen. As they are in this house of
mud, so they have to start with this house of mud, with the
conquest of the body. The body should not be your enemy;
it should not be the one that dictates to you; you are the
one who dictates to the body, breaking some of its habits.
All of this comes under the category of tapas—heating up,
exertion, changing the habit by doing something over and
over again.

In ancient and medieval times there were certain
undesirable schools of teaching among whom tapas or
asceticism was so extreme that it was unpleasant both to
the doer and the viewer. On the other hand in the
nineteenth and twentieth centuries, we have seen an
extreme reaction against that kind of asceticism. Just as a
goal of a religious mind in the fourteenth, fifteenth, or
sixteenth centuries was to reach God by purification
through this kind of unpleasant asceticism, the goal of the
modern person is comfort. Extreme asceticism has given
way to extreme comfort. Now, what hatha yoga is, is
comfortable asceticism. Do not make yourself too uncomfortable, and yet exert a little. If you do it harmoniously

and gently, your purpose will be accomplished. Gradually you will become comfortable with it, and perhaps uncomfortable without it. So this is a milder form of physical asceticism historically. And, again, it is practiced for the purpose of the conquest of the body.

Why this conquest of the body? Take, for example, the Christian doctrine of the conquest of the flesh. When the phrase "master of flesh" is used in the West, immediately the thought goes to questions like mastering sexual desire or some other desire. But, here, we are not talking merely of mastering one desire as against another but of mastering all the functions of the entire body as a whole—every function. While you are practicing postures, for that duration, there is no other desire. Why? Because the mind can desire only one thing at a time, and for the duration of, say, forty-five minutes you have set your mind to watch the body developing, becoming relaxed, releasing tensions, removing its pain and so on until the body is so trained that it learns to obey the mind. A person who practices hatha yoga regularly, daily, will have an easier time mastering the desires of the flesh than a person who does not. Here we are not speaking of a puritanical ideal; we are not turning everyone into lifelong celibates. As another example, take the desire to overeat: when you are sensitive to the body, it is much easier to conquer such a desire. You learn how to absorb your energies into your system and reuse them.

This conquest by the mind of the body, then, is the first philosophical goal of hatha yoga: that the body should be under the direction of the mind. The mind says, "Move." The body moves. The mind says, "Rise without touching your hand to the ground, just using your calf muscles, knees, and thigh muscles." The body does so. The body does not say, "Oh, I feel so slothful, I think I'll just lie here in this comfortable bed surrounded with these comfortable cushions on this horrible spine-twisting mattress. I am so comfortable." That kind of powerless power that the body has over the mind has to be broken. Otherwise you can neither sit in meditation for a long time, nor can you breathe deeply, nor can you stay healthy, nor can you run your digestive system in any kind of proper order.

To make the body a fit vessel for God's worship becomes the purpose of hatha yoga. That was the purpose, the only reason, for which the ancient yogis started the science of hatha yoga. If the body is not purified, then it will have adverse effects on the processes of mental purification. Sooner or later, one place or another, the body will become a hindrance to the mind in its own practice of worship, prayer, or meditation. This tapas, this exertion, this gentle exertion, is where the entire practice of hatha yoga fits in with the teaching of the great master, Patanjali.

The second aspect of hatha yoga is its relationship to worship. It is difficult to determine how many people practicing physical yoga are devotionally minded. But to me, hatha yoga is worship. And in this I am not inventing something or making up a new interpretation. The interpretation itself has always existed because that is what it was when the entire practice was begun. It is only in the modern context, both in India and the West, that hatha has become separated from worship. Modern man knows worship only with speech: sing a hymn, recite a prayer, utter inspiring words, and so on., Worship with the body and worship with the mind, these two aspects, have been almost completely forgotten.

Now, a truth-seeker is one in whom mind, speech, and body all act together, in unison. In fact, in the ancient tradition, one of the definitions of personal truth, in terms of truthful speech and truthful acts, is that "What one thinks with the mind, that one utters with the speech; what one utters with the speech, that one puts into action; what one thus puts into action is accomplished and fulfilled." The entire personality is involved. And likewise with hatha yoga, neither worship nor exercise should, then, be separated from each other. The muscles, the mouth, the mind—everything—*must* be involved.

This integration of the entire personality can be experienced with *surya-namaskara,* the solar salutation. In India, it was and is a tradition that for the morning and evening worship, one sits facing the sun. In the Christian tradition, the sun is a symbol of Christ; sunrise is Easter. We have all of these symbolic associations. All worship in India is performed not only facing the sun but, if possible, facing other beautiful, natural phenomena. For example, sitting by a river, sitting by flowing waters, and meditating is a most beautiful experience.

Sun is the symbol of light. The ideal is to wake up before sunrise. In India, people normally walk out of the village before sunrise and do their morning ablutions in the flowing water. Now, it is not possible elsewhere always because of such a great fluctuation of seasons. But in India, the fluctuation is not more than an hour or so. The morning hour from 4:30 a.m. or even an hour or so earlier is regarded as *brahma-muhurta,* the hour of Brahman, the godly hour.

The *brahma-muhurta,* that hour from 3 a.m. to 4:30 a.m. or so, is a very strange, a very powerful hour. A great number of violent crimes are committed at that hour. A great many deaths in the hospitals are reported to occur at that hour. A large number of conceptions occur at that hour. It is an hour when the energy field around us is more intense. It is the natural hour for worship, for tapas, for any kind of practice. You can warp your energies and commit violent crimes or you can fall in love and be instrumental in the occurrence of a conception or you can sit up and do your meditation at that hour.

Now, not all yogis meditate at this time, but in a large majority of ashrams in India, that is the hour people wake up, maintain a certain attitude, take a shower, and do their practice. This should not be taken legalistically, because people will say, "Well, I cannot get up a 4 a.m., so I don't think I am going to practice any more hatha." That is not the idea. But in the early morning hour you can stand facing the rising sun. In fact, the word for "worship" in the Sanskrit language, *sandhya,* also means dawn or dusk, a junction, a conjunction of the day and the night.

When you stand before the sun, you should not stand just before an ordinary natural phenomenon. The whole process of yoga depends on the philosophical realization of one fact that we have spoken of repeatedly: the correspondence between the microcosm (the small world of the personality) and the macrocosm (the universe). What is in this egg, the roughly oval outline of the body in a meditative posture, is in the cosmic egg. Whatever is in the cosmic egg is in this egg also. The idea in yoga (*yoga =* yoke, join) is to establish the connection between the two, to unite the two.

As the sun and the moon shine out there, where are the sun and the moon within me? Why is it that my blood is called to the seashore? What is the connection between my arteries and veins and the rivers flowing on this earth? The light and the splendor that I see over there is the light and the splendor that is in my eyes; and the light and the splendor that is in my eyes does not exist of its own accord but because of another light known as the light of prana in my mind, the light of prana and vitality in my system. The sun represents the prana within. There is one text on the subject of prana that should be read, one of the eleven principal Upanishads, the Prashna Upanishad.

What is the connection of prana, this inner vitality, with the sun that shines? It is not only that we receive an awakening, an awareness of the rays of the physical sun, but that the very thing that shines in the sun, that very force that is the prana and vitality and awareness and aliveness in our systems—those two things are one and the same with the Divine Light. It is the same one light that shines in both, and that is why the two are mutually attracted. It is not that both of them have a common origin but rather that both of them are one. And when you look at the sun, it should immediately remind you of the great light shining like ten thousand suns that the great meditation masters have reported of their own experiences of inner realization, because everything external is a symbol for whatever is internal. There should never be any external act in your life which is not somewhere connected internally with the divine figure in you.

Doing the morning hatha is physically establishing that relationship. You come out and stand before the sun and look up—but you don't just start, you let go of your body and immerse yourself in that field of light: the spiritual light within, the light of prana in your vitality, in your physical personality, the light of the sun in the whole universe. You establish that mental contact. Without that, your attitude is not right and you cannot begin to do yoga, because yoga is union. When you are doing hatha yoga and start with the solar salutation, what is the union? Whose union with whom? Unification of the principle of the entire

sun salutation

field of light, the mental light, the light of the sun. Stand there before the sun and it becomes, for you, symbolic of your object of worship. "Here the sun rises and shines within me"—and immediately the body and mind should become filled with prana. You cannot do anything but get into a worshipful attitude.

The *chakra* of prayer is the *anahata chakra*. Yes, the center of consciousness for devotion and prayer is the heart center. Now, a lot of people bring their hands together thinking, "Well, we are supposed to join hands; what effect does it have on the hands; what benefit do I get by joining the hands? Does it strengthen the wrist or does it strengthen the fingers?" If one looks for only those kinds of external benefits, one is not going to get far in the practice of hatha yoga. When the solar salutation is taught, we are

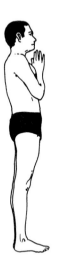

told that the ridges of the thumbs are held against the cardiac center. A gentle pressure is applied; the emotional center is released. You are conscious of a humble, devout attitude arising within you, and when you apply this pressure in the cardiac area, immediately it has the effect of inclining you to bend the neck and bow the head. And that physical feeling is not simply a physical reaction but a worshipful attitude. Only after you have felt that, and then straightened up, do your exercises begin.

This is not something peculiar to the practice of hatha yoga. The Indian classical dancing always begins with a chant, with an homage, with a passage of worship, surrender. Dancing was developed in the temples because it was, again, an act of worshiping with the body. They worshiped with the body and enacted the stories of the great incarnations in the dance form. The thought of dance as part of, let us say, a Christmas Mass is something that may seem peculiar here. Yet in worshiping Krishna in India, for example, one would not dream of devotion without some kind of a dance step, a worship with the body. Worship is not something you do only with the mouth, only with speech.

So hatha yoga is worship with the body, and each gesture has a mental connection. Join the hands in the shape of a not-quite-blooming flower and the bud opens up and becomes a flower, and this is the symbol of a flower. This flower is placed before the heart center. Every secret fragrance of a flower out there in the world is in my heart waiting to be exuded as the fragrance of my prayer, my worship, my devotion looking for something great.

If one does not wish to name that something great "God," one can name it the sun, or the Supreme Being, or the consciousnesss force. Name it whatever you wish—an internal river, if you wish—but the attitude of worship is important to beginning the practice of hatha. One naturally wants to rise and face the sun. I rise up to you; I open my eyes to you; I open my arms to you; I go there and I am so taken up, my soul, my spirit, is so carried upward with your magnificence, I feel so humble, so modest, so little, that I bow down.

The first movement of the solar salutation is my opening

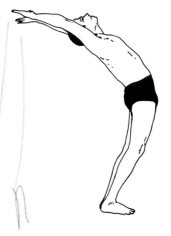

the eyes, opening the arms, rising up, facing the sun, feeling the prana come, the great magnificence of the *Brhat,* the vast life force shining before me, my arms reaching out to the whole universe, to touch with the light in my fingers the light that shines in all the galaxies. And when I reach there and touch the magnificence, it is so great, and I feel so very small that I bow down; my hands go down to the very earth, and I touch the earth with my hands—that solid earth I am standing on, that light, that magnificence, that power; prana has come here, and it is also rising within me from within the earth. I touch the solid earth; I stretch down, my head is down to my knees, and I see all creation; I see not only angels and *devas* and gods and incarnations but also the ordinary living beings, those who are on four feet. With them also I establish communion; 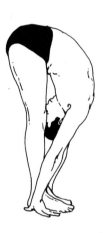 I see this earth the way they see it; the way the earth sustains them sustains me also, and so for the moment I go along with them and lovingly share this.

The entire series of movements is this poetic hymn of the body. If your mind is not in tune with the mood of that poetic hymn, there is no hatha yoga—*ha,* the sun, *tha,* the moon. Both the sun and the moon should be present there—the light, and the coolness; the exertion, and the relaxation; that which is internal, and, that which is external; that which is self-luminous, and that which shines by reflected light—besides all of the technical jargon of trying to balance the breaths in the right and left nostrils and so on. If a person recites this cosmic poetry with his body in the morning, he will experience the full enjoyment

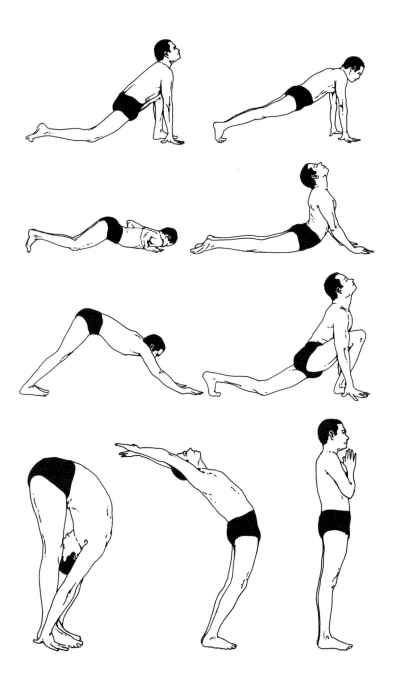

of hatha yoga. That is worship. The entire series of exercises should be done with that kind of an attitude. One goes through the series of postures and feels what each is a symbol of—what attitude it conveys. Even the names of the various exercises are significant.

Many people do not know that in the ancient tradition this entire process was part of the worship ritual. Even now, people who practice no hatha yoga go through this daily morning ritual, this poetry rising from the heart. A traditional Indian chalice, or *kalasha,* is a water jar shaped like a person's head used for bathing, to carry holy water, and so forth, as well as to make devotional offerings of water. And right from the very beginning a child is taught to take the vessel full of water— full, never empty—down to the river in the morning to sit and meditate, after bathing. A person takes this full vessel of water—always fullness, symbolic of 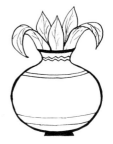 a human head full of thoughts, or, on the emotional level, of what a human being most cherishes as a child: mother's breast—and sits with this full vessel of water. Never emptiness, always fullness. Sometimes, if he wants to pray for a sick person, he places his hands on this full vessel of water while he sits in meditation. In his mind at the end of meditation, he surrenders the fruit of that meditation with a healing prayer for that person and gives him the water to drink or sprinkles the water on him as a healing touch.

After the morning meditation under a tree, on the grass, by the river, one brings that full vessel of water home. The vessel is never carried home empty. Historically, it was thought that if someone was leaving for a trip and a friend brought a full vessel of water, it was a very good omen; it was symbolic of having a good journey. Fullness was always emphasized. Sometimes a few blades of grass or a few green leaves would be placed in it before walking home. In fact, even in the modern languages of India, asking somebody "Are you well?" is "Are you *kushala*?" The word *kushala* literally means "he who brings something green in the morning after worship," which means, in turn, "Are you well enough mentally to wake up in the morning and go out and do your meditational worship, well enough to walk all that way, balanced enough to remember to pick something green and put it in that full water vessel and bring it home?" All of that is involved in the word *kushala*. Are you *kushala*? Are you well?

Sometimes a child is taught to go and fill the vessel with water and stand before the sun and pour an offering of waters in a steady stream and watch that steady stream, letting the breath flow with that steady stream of water.

These are all symbols. Some of the acts in the hatha exercises are symbolic. The movement of the arm is an offering of your arm to the Divine: it is not simply to build a muscle, but "Here, I give to you my arm; I receive from you strength and movement." A forward movement with an exhalation going down is a gesture of humility, modesty, bending down toward Mother Earth; and a movement upward, backwards, is looking upward at the sky, filling myself with the sun, with the light, thinking of that light which is in me here and coming into contact with that cosmic magnificence; and, again, coming back to earth and exhaling. Holding a posture, holding still, means maintaining there what you have filled yourself with.

In the universe, all cycles, all spirals, go in a series of creation, maintenance, and dissolution. All worship in this tradition is an enactment of the universal cycles: creation, maintenance, and dissolution—the trinity of Brahma, Vishnu, Shiva; Creator, Preserver, Destroyer. In the asanas also is that creation, maintenance, and then going back through the cycle. The cycle of the asanas should remind you of this cycle of expiration-death, inspiration-birth, and maintenance: the cycle of birth and death and reincarnation. Holding the posture longer symbolizes lengthening the life span; it also actually effects the prolongation of life.

The first thing in the morning is a bowel movement. A child is trained for that from the very beginning—emptying, cleansing. One cannot do exercises with the bowels full. Washing the mouth, taking a shower, doing the physical yoga, sitting down. Physical yoga naturally moves into relaxation; relaxation naturally moves into meditation. If your body is fit and your inner parts are clean, your mind will not be oppressed. Then you naturally go out into the world and have an extremely happy day. You sing all day wherever you are. Some of the boys in the ashram help me by driving me here and there sometimes, and the girls say, "You get this opportunity of being with Panditji." And the boys say, "No, all he does is sit in the car and either meditates or sings." But I'm just happy. There are very, very few reasons in my life to be unhappy. Enjoy yourself. There is a phrase in the Hindi language: *khush raho*—be happy; stand there, laugh at the wind.

There is a stipulation in India's Constitution that certain arts and cultural activities have to be represented in the Upper House (like the U.S. Senate). A very famous actor, Prithiviraj, was given this honor. Once he was questioned about the secret of his success with reference to a role he had played, portraying Lord Krishna in the

Bhagavad Gita. He replied, "The secret of my success? I do not know any secret. But when I was playing this role of Lord Krishna, at that time I was not on stage; I was five thousand years back in that battlefield and I was Krishna. It was as if the spirit of Krishna had overtaken my entire personality and my mind and was speaking through me. It was the most spiritual, most meditative experience of my life—to stand there and be filmed. I was not aware of those cameras. To be filmed speaking and teaching Arjuna; here was a seeker aspiring." And this is the secret with hatha yoga. The hatha yoga itself can liberate you.

So there is this awareness in each posture; in each posture there should be this interpretation from the heart: a prayer, a worship, an awareness. When I place my body in that posititon, what mood naturally evolves? Or, what mood would make me place myself in such a position? It can be looked at both ways. What mood induces such a body position, and what mood does such a body position invoke? You can experiment; you know your body, you know its language, you know what it means when you are "like this" and what it means when you are "like that." So what is the connection of that mood, that thought, with the posture. Observe it, analyze it, and conquer it.

The conquest of mood means that in your life you are never subject to the tyranny of moods, that your moods are subject to your pleasure. Do you know the tyranny of moods? "I can't do this because I'm not in the mood. I am down and depressed." How can we be down and depressed when we woke up in the morning and looked at the sun and raised our eyes to the galaxies, took that light into our bodies and brought it down to the very earth? And from that earth, we rose again and looked up and resurrected ourselves. How can we be down and depressed for the rest of the day? It is not enough for us to just sit there with our shoulders down and say we are like the light of the sun, but rather we must go through the postures and cultivate the attitude of strength and conquest. Not only conquest of the body but conquest of moods is what hatha yoga will accomplish for you.

There is no reason for one to go to a psychiatrist. Depressed? Okay, snap out of it. That's what is done in hatha: you place yourself in all kinds of possible positions and then observe yourself. What would the world be like if I were not standing on my two feet and did not have my two hands—if I were a cobra? What then would be my interpretation of the world? You get into the cobra pose and see the world as a cobra sees it. You become the master of your incarnations. You remember all your evolutionary stages. Then you say, "No . . . this is fine as a cobra, but I do not want to remain a cobra. One good thing I have learned from the cobra is to feel the strength in my spinal muscles and the fullness of the breath in my chest. Now I rise up again." In a single hatha session you pass through the entire cycle of reincarnation, pass through the entire cycle of having been a tree, a locust, a fish, a crocodile, a cobra, an eagle, a camel, a lion, a child, a warrior, a corpse, and the entire cycle of creation, preservation, and destruction. Every day, creation of a mood, preservation of that mood, and removal of that mood to something else can be accomplished at your will. A dancer will tell you that true dance comes from the mood. You create the mood and then become that.

This leads us to hatha yoga as a burning of karma.

3

Karma Purification

One of the purposes of hatha yoga is the burning of karma. Yoga philosophy believes that nothing happens in the body without its first happening in the mind. Nothing whatsoever. You sow certain seeds in your mental personality. You drop a seed in the soil of your mind, where it grows; it becomes either a mango tree or a mulberry bush, poison ivy or a rose, whichever one you wish to sow. If you sow a rose, it is a rose that grows from you. You have placed in your mind the raw material of your thought. Each thought once placed in the mind becomes the raw material for a further thought. For example, the very sentence you have just read has now been placed in your mind. Its impression having been stored in the mind becomes the raw material for a subsequent thought. Some other thoughts will arise out of it, consciously or unconsciously, directly or indirectly, depending on how much this seed-thought is watered, how much you contemplate it, how much you strengthen it. Every act you perform with your body is a thought. Every act you perform with your speech, too, is a thought planted in your mind.

This is where hatha yoga and meditation connect.

Every act a person performs with his body is a thought planted in his mind. So it is a new karma, a new act being planted in the mind. A person plants lazy thoughts in his mind every time he slouches. That lazy thought becomes the seed or raw material for a further thought. So it becomes a habit. So he lies comfortably on a pillow and does not want to get up for the next morning's asanas. And when he finally does get up it is too late, and hungry or not hungry, by force of habit he reaches for the mother's breast, or a substitute called the refrigerator, to gain emotional security and treat himself to a surrogate suck-ling. That is the psychology of unnecessary eating. And we all do this sort of thing continuously.

Whenever people ask me what they should do to stop themselves from overeating, I immediatley say to find out what their emotional frustrations are. When the mind is deadened and unfulfilled, a person fills his stomach to the full and thinks that thereby he is fulfilling the mind. By fulfilling the mind in the stomach he thinks he is filling the mind in the mind. So he decides to eat at the wrong time in the wrong way, and sit in a wrong way and think in a wrong way while eating. The previous meal is not yet digested, but he puts more in there. He decides to do this.

This process of wrong decision making eventually becomes the cause of a disease. So disease is then a ripening of the poison ivy plant from the seed planted in the original lazy thought, the original attitude of sloth-fulness which becomes a thought, which then gives him the decision to remain lazy, not to use the body correctly, not to use the food properly, not to use sleep in the right way. And then that suffering becomes the fruition of his kar-ma and he later complains of having so much suffering. The instrument of discrimination, the *buddhi,* becomes occluded by cloudy thoughts and gets into the wrong process of decision making, and thereby one makes choices to use the body wrongfully. The natural karmic result of these poor decisions is suffering, which is really only a purging of accumulated toxins and such. The body has built up deposit after deposit of poison, so it has to express itself or get it out through colds or the flu or diarrhea or acne or something or the other; salt deposits or mineral deposits or calcium deposits or cancer.

What the hatha yogis do is follow a very wise principle, which has been spoken of by all the schools of wisdom and philosophy in the whole world and which is one of the many secrets of a happy life. This principle is that whatever you dislike, do voluntarily and willingly, if you do not want it to come to you by force. Whatever you do not like, do voluntarily. Whatever you are running away from, turn and face it squarely and say, "What is it that I am afraid of? Let me examine you. Let me analyze this fear, this horrible thing that I dread, this terrible thing I do not like coming to me, that I run away from."

For instance, a natural instinct of every dog going to sleep at night in the wilds is to find a nice leafy area to make itself comfortable; similarly it is the habit of every lazy body like mine and yours to find a nice cushion or quilt, and so on. We are running away from physical discomfort. The idea behind tapas, asceticism, is to take voluntarily what you otherwise absolutely dislike. Turn around and say, "Let's see, now, what is this discomfort that I run away from?" At every step you do that in your life. If you want to attain perfection—perfection in health, perfection in mind, perfection in speech, perfection in action, perfection in spirituality, perfection in godliness—whatever you are running away from, find out what it is and turn around and look at it straight in the eyes and examine it. As soon as you will turn around, this thing that you have feared for so long will try to run away from you. If you run away from it, it chases you, but as soon as you turn around and say, "Hey, now you have found me," it tries to run away. You tell it, "You have been chasing me and I have been running away from you. Now you better stand right here. Let me examine you. What is your anatomy? What is it that I fear?" Examine that. Analyze it.

So in hatha yoga there is the same principle, that this love of physical comfort, wrongly interpreted, is slothfulness, negligence, laziness, all of that. That is to be removed. And we turn around, and where in the body the mind's actions have deposited fat and blubber and many other unnecessary things, we remove them as a voluntary act of karma purification. We can take fifteen minutes of daily discomfort or we can take fifteen days in a hospital. The choice is ours. If we do not pay the karma voluntarily, then it will be paid involuntarily; then fifteen years from now we will spend fifteen months in the hospital. It is entirely our choice. The karma must be paid. If we will not put ourselves on a diet, the doctor will put us on one. If we will not do it today, we will have to do it fifteen years from now and then we will come face to face with the whole accumulation, and we will have to handle it.

So part of the practice of hatha yoga is to make up for karma, to take a little physical discomfort of our own choice so that the seeds we have sown in the soil of our minds come to fruition and get paid off very quickly. The fat on the body is only a symbol of the fat in the mind. It is an expression of the occlusion of the mind. It is an expression of wrong decision making at every step, at every moment.

In the Yoga Sutras, the purification exercises are called *shaucha,* the first of the five *niyamas. Shaucha* is a word both for physical cleanliness and mental purity. As the mind aspires for purity it immediately becomes conscious of the unclean things in the body. A clean, clear mind is a pure mind, a yogically purified mind. By a clear mind, I do not mean one clear on a certain subject; rather, the mind itself is entirely clear, or clarified.

The mind in which there is no occlusion becomes very conscious of all its surroundings, very sensitive to them. A yogi in meditation becomes aware of all the poisons in the lymph nodes. As I mentioned earlier, he is sensitive to even the slightest particle of material in the colon. He is aware of factors about which an average individual is not concerned. I have observed very carefully the effect of food on meditation. I have to eat at all different times because I fix my time of eating according to the meditations I have to conduct—at what hour, and how much space I need to keep between them—because as soon as the food goes into the stomach, I immediately notice it, as an occlusion of the prana force. It takes a number of different types of exercises (subtle internal exercises, not physical exercises) to clear the mind of that occlusion that comes from the intake of food.

So we go from purification of the mind, automatically, to purification of the body. A pure mind cannot live in an impure body, just as a clear mind cannot live in confused surroundings. A clear mind has fixed daily habits. For example, a very unhealthy habit is that of eating in the morning without having had a bowel movement. It is unthinkable for any person aspiring for health. How can one continue to pile more food on top of digested food which needs to be eliminated? By practicing *shaucha,* purification of mind, a person will become naturally inclined to purification of the body.

What is the relationship between the physical body and the subtle body? We have said that nothing happens in the physical body without something first happening in the subtle body. It is inconceivable for me to be able to smell a flower unless the smell principle is first in the consciousness; it is inconceivable to touch something solid unless first the abstract principle of the consciousness of solidity is present in the mind. Or else the two—the subject and the object—would not connect. An object would be there, but the subject would not be aware of it. Just as it applies to this external personality in reaction to the objects around it, it applies even more so to the relationship between the subtle body and the objects around it. What is the object around the subtle body? The physical body. What is the object around the self? The mind. What are the objects around the subtle body? Hands, feet, legs, and organs. What are the objects around the physical body? Walls, tape recorders, and all the rest. So what applies to a relationship between the stimulus from the objects and response from the senses also applies to stimulus from the physical body into the subtle body, and the response of the subtle body onto the physical body.

What are many physicians doing today? They give their patients pills to take care of their thyroid problems. But from what karma, what kind of consciousness, does that thyroid problem arise? This is not being considered. So the symptoms are being suppressed. But as to the mental aspect, the karmic aspect, nothing is being done about it. The root cause of the symptom is not dealt with.

This is true today in the West not only about medicine, but even about the areas of psychology. For instance, why are there such sudden explosions of interest in astrology? For the same reason that so many people go to psychiatrists. It is just another symptom of current emotional insecurity—"What will the future be like? What will happen? What will happen to me?" If a person doesn't have a mother or a father, he has a psychiatrist; or if he doesn't have a psychiatrist, then he has an astrologer. A lot of people not recognizing this fact and interested in these areas will possibly be offended by this statement, but ninety-nine percent of the people who come to see me and who are interested in astrology are just exhibiting signs of emotional instability and feelings of insecurity. They worry about the future and have an absence of faith and confidence in themselves—looking to the stars for guidance.

In India, where the science of astrology has reached a degree of perfection and is used so commonly, there exists this feeling of insecurity also. However, the astrologers in India always view it in a karmic context. They say, "This and this is coming your way, but you can ward it off by doing such and such karma, or undertaking such and such practice, or making such and such charity." They say, for example, "Go and buy three yards of red cloth and give it to somebody" or "Buy so many kilos of sesame seeds and give them to someone." Give such and such kind of charity to ward off such and such kind of situation which is expected to develop in your life. Whether it is the act itself, or the thought behind it, whatever is there, there is something karmic about it; and there is knowledge that you are capable of warding off these influences around you.

So, through a change of mind, through a change in the subtle body, you remove the causes for, say, that thyroid problem. You work on the mental level. You give some-body a mantra which goes with concentration on the throat center, and you teach him to do the shoulderstand. A mantra, a concentration, a shoulderstand, and then you say, "Continue with your prescribed medicine until you overcome the need for it." Nothing happens to a person's throat unless he has some warp of energy in his subtle body. Thus you work from the physical angle, and also from the energy angle. Work on them together and you have treatment of the whole being—the physical being, the being in the subtle body, the being in the mind—on the meditational level, on the karmic level, and so on. It is a long-term process. Modern Western medicine is designed for quick results, and it relieves the pain very quickly, but usually only temporarily. All things considered, I doubt that even with modern technology the sum total of pain on this planet has been reduced, taking into account emo-tional pain, physical pain, family pain, and so on.

People often ask me about auras. They ask, "What color is my aura?" and so forth. Few people in the East or the West know anything about auras. The aura of an individual—whatever it is that is called an aura—differs from emotion to emotion, differs from moment to moment; just as the reading of a palm is nothing reliable, because the palm changes every six months as one changes his mind. I have watched my palm; I make a new decision and the lines of the palm change. On the other hand, weak-minded people are beguiled; an astrologer says, "You will commit suicide at the age of eighteen," so the person goes and commits suicide at the age of eighteen. But what was the cause and what was the effect? Maybe the statement itself was the cause of the person's commiting suicide. Things should always be approached from a standpoint of strength, not weakness. A strong-minded person is not affected by such prophesies. He may see the trends through astrology and palmistry, but by the application of his will he gives them a new direction. A man of God says: "Who guides my life? The stars? Who guides the stars? God. I will let my free will and life be guided by the one who guides the stars." This is *ishvara-pranidhana,* surrender to God, faith, the fifth *niyama* among the eight limbs of yoga.

Now the question is of practice, living by the letter of the law, so to speak, rather than by the spirit. Quite often people are doing their practices legally and mechanically: "It is prescribed, 'Thou shalt move thy arm at such and such an angle,' so I shall move my arm at such and such an angle." But their overall attitude to life is not changing. This is seen in the craze about diets, and substituting one kind of drug culture for another kind of drug culture, and yet the overall attitude about diet is not changing. Food still remains an object that is picked up and put in the mouth when one craves it or when one gets hungry. A person experiments with diet and says, "I am going to eat raw fruit only." But when he eats it or how he eats it or how much he eats of it is ignored. He also ignores the idea of gratefully accepting the gift of food and passing on this gift by offering food to someone else. He eats it without offering it to anybody else. There are two people sharing an apartment and there is one apple. The person who comes into the apartment first picks up the apple, eats it, finishes it. That's not diet. Leave half for the other person and keep half the stomach empty. That is the yoga idea of revolution in diet—sharing with love.

Then the individual mind will draw into the individual body the cosmic prana. I see young people—sixteen, seventeen, eighteen years old—running to doctors every day. They are trying all kinds of diets, and the more they go to the doctor, the more sick they are, because the mind reinforces the idea, "I'm sick, I'm sick." So the sickness comes, the mind brings out all of that sickness. This is not to say that you shouldn't go to the doctor if you are sick! Please, that is not what I mean.

What I am saying is that we cannot take one little thing in isolation and experiment with it without changing our whole karma about it, without making it part of our overall growth. I would rather have a person eat meat, and share it, than become a vegetarian, live on the diet of a hermit, and not share his food with others in mind. If you eat only for your own indulgence, says the Bhagavad Gita (III:13), you eat only sin.

People ask, "Should I take a shower before my hatha yoga, or after my hatha yoga?" They expect to have a prescribed law. But what is a shower? If we cannot revive the concept that all waters are mother waters, that going to the water is going to the womb, taking a dip in the primeval, cosmic ocean, that taking a daily shower is Jesus being baptized in the river Jordan, that taking a shower is an act of renunciation, an act of washing off the dirt of the body and of the mind—if that attitude is not there, whether we take a shower before or after doing hatha postures (or even at all) isn't going to matter much. It's going to keep our bodies clean, and that's all. But its overall psychological impact is being missed—because we have demolished mythology, because we have killed Milton, because we have murdered Dante, because we have destroyed the ancient Greek culture, because we have cut off our connections between the individual mind and the cosmic mind, because we are too ashamed to recite poetry in school. Because of all those collective, cultural murders, entering a shower is for us only washing the dirt and sweat from the body; but the psychological satisfaction, the spiritual satisfaction, the ritual satisfaction, the washing of the mind, changing the overall pattern of thought—that is missing.

That is where the basic psychological problems of the modern person are; the objects are just objects and have no psychic connections. There is nothing from the subtle body flowing between ourselves and the mother waters. Unless this overall attitude changes, just moving the body in the sun salutation is of no use. Rather, when we practice our physical yoga, let our connection of the mind be between the core of the mind and the vast field of cosmic energy. The two are one.

In yoga philosophy there are three universal qualities: *tamas* (stability), *rajas* (activity), and *sattva* (harmony). On the personal level tamas may take the form of lethargy, heaviness of mind, or depression; rajas may take the form of excitement or nervousness; and sattva may take the form of joyfulness, clarity of mind, and calmness. Everything in nature has these three qualities. Food does also, and, as with all things in his environment, a yogi is selective about what he allows himself to experience because each experience leaves its impression on the subtle body.

Certain foods are tamasic, or sattvic, or rajasic, but more than that *we* are sattvic, or rajasic, or tamasic. Eating should be viewed in its overall context. Fine, choose the right food. But let us choose the right attitude that goes with the food. Otherwise, that right food becomes wrong food. If instead of eating meat we eat salad, but we serve only ourselves, we have planted a seed of karma which will bring digestive problems. Digestive problems arise karmically from selfish eating. So, selfish eating creates in the mind the condition whereby those kinds of anxieties will arise in us and we will have ulcers. It is good to eat sattvic food, but better still to have a sattvic disposition while eating it. If in a past life we have spoken only lies, we have kept a secret sin that has kept us tense and anxious, we cannot help but have asthma. (Of course this is not the only cause of this illness; all diseases develop from a variety of reasons, but we are speaking here only what is relevant to the present discussion.)

We can overcome that condition karmically by undertaking certain types of action—fresh actions to counter those psychological effects from the subtle body. But it cannot be done with a guilt feeling; it can be done only with positive reinforcement. So if I say, "I am suffering from digestive problems, and this is from the karma of selfish eating; so from now on when I prepare a salad I'll always go and knock at the next door apartment and share my salad so that I will stop suffering from digestive problems," that's not going to work. "Let me look for a monk who has a begging bowl. Let me send a few bananas to the Himalayan Institute so I will stop having digestive problems." No, this approach will not do. There has to be the intent to love, to be concerned, to share—and it has to be pure, positive, altruistic, without seeking results therefrom, without asking for fruits of that action. Only then will it bring the necessary changes in the subtle body, which will very minutely adjust the relationship between the mental body and the physical body. That minute, intangible adjustment will change the flow of secretions in our glands and will begin to undo the damage caused by the warping of energies due to past selfishness.

Besides changing the energy pattern of the subtle body by altering one's attitude and conduct, there are other ways to help remedy diseases. The hatha exercises can be done mentally for persons who are so sick that they cannot move through them. The exercises are done for the ailing part of the body mentally. But there is one secret. That is breath. For example, if you have an ulcer, lie in your bed, relax your whole body, and exhale as if the malignancy of the ulcer is being exhaled out from that point, out through the path of the breath. If you have a boil on the body, you can do the same. It will reduce your pain and it will reduce some of the poisons. It is the breath that is flowing from that point upward, outward through the nostrils—then inhale as if peace and healing are going down to that point. If you have a problem and you cannot take exercise now, you can take breathing exercises—breathing as if the breath is flowing out from the cardiac area and flowing upward, and flowing into that area. Do it for a good one hour every day lying in bed at home or in the hospital. This is the first exercise in the complex and long art of self-healing.

At the same time we are also working from the physical angle, doing our exercise with this openness of the heart. When we are opening our arms, we shouldn't just open our arms out into empty space; we are opening our arms out to the whole universe. When we close our arms, it is not a selfish act of drawing in, but embracing and gathering. We shouldn't let hatha yoga become an actor's theatrical performance. Let the positive mood arise. The greatest problem in the practice of hatha yoga, or an artist practicing his art, is that the mood does not change at his command. And that is one thing that we need to learn—to change our moods at that time and not just give a demonstration of physical acrobatics. So whether it is taking a bath or opening our arms, let that be a trigger to the mind.

∴ Be mindful — always

There are, for example, certain mantras that go with different movements of the sun salutation. There is one whole mantra that goes through twenty-five cycles of the sun salutation. Certain mantras are practiced in certain positions. Also, the various names of the asanas, animal names, refer to karmic cycles. A basic series of eighty-four asanas has historically been taught, symbolizing a cycle of eighty-four hundred thousand species and subspecies through which the soul has made a journey to become a human being. And those eighty-four asanas represent titles, one for every one hundred thousand. I'm not in a position to enumerate all the eighty-four hundred thousand species and subspecies; but the seekers went into the positions and realized, "Here too is life. What can I learn from a snake? What can I learn from a camel's body?" For example, the upper wash is called *kunjala kriya,* "the act of the elephant." An elephant takes in a certain amount of water and then spews it out, so the ancient yogis also took water in and learned to spew it out every morning to wash the stomach. The yogis observed all the animals and said, "Now, what are the healthy things they do instinctively that we, in our intellectualism, have forgotten?" They watched the snake stretch itself and saw what effect it would have (a snake is nothing but a spine). The practice of *trataka,* gazing, was learned by observing snakes, too, because there are certain species of snakes said to hypnotize their victims. (Whether they hypnotize the victims or whether the victims looking at them become hypnotized with fear is another matter.)

When a seeker practiced an asana, he reestablished a relationship between the instinctive and the intellectual. If the entire science of hatha yoga and asanas were lost completely today, sooner or later humanity would rediscover it—some persons who were sensitive to themselves and to the animal kingdom would find its knowledge within themselves. There is something instinctive in nature, in our nature, crying out to expand, to be expounded, to be used.

I was amazed when I first brought my newborn son, Angiras, home from the hospital. Infants are born breathing diaphragmatically. Have you ever watched a baby breathe—how his whole trunk moves? Here I am sending instructors out all over to teach people diaphragmatic breathing, and the students are paying out so much in fees to learn to breathe diaphragmatically. "My boy, where did you learn this? What school of yoga did you go to?" So in a human being there is this natural yoga. What is a yawn? Carbon dioxide builds up, the body wants oxygen, there is tension, the body wants release; so we do a hatha yoga stretch, a yawn, natural hatha.

If we observe our natural inclinations, there is a certain point where the whole yoga practice will come to us. We have to learn it now by prescription because we are not sensitive to whatever is natural in us. Why? Because we have been incorrectly trained in the use of the mind; we have been told that the rational mind is the only worthwhile mind. We have been taught that what does not appeal to the rational mind is worthless: discard it, throw it away: religion, ritual, mythology, sensitivity, environment, instinct, everything—throw it away. In the process, what women of the primitive tribes of Africa practice naturally at childbirth, here we have to go to classes to learn. Dr. Leboyer observed the women of India at childbirth and wrote his book, which is selling in the millions. So: self-sensitivity, self-observation; an overall view of the universe—where we are in that universe, what our connections are, how the energy, the flickers of our minds are related to the flickers in the corona of the sun—observe that the two are one and the same movement. We know this in the moon and in the tides and in the menstrual cycles, yet we don't understand it.

The real philosophy of hatha yoga can come to us by practice, practice of the mind—doing it as a mental exercise, as an act of worship, as an act of reestablishing the relationship both with the lower world and with the higher world: the lower world of the instincts, of the snake and the camel and the elephant; and the higher world of the beings of energy which we really are—beings of energy which have come and occupied these physical bodies and are exercising control over them. In that context, we should practice our yoga and enjoy it. We should enjoy it fully and not make it a chore.

The relationship between hatha yoga and meditation comes at four points. Where does hatha yoga leave off and meditation begin? Of course, hatha yoga itself is a meditative practice; but then there are four areas of transition, four links between hatha yoga and meditation proper. You do your set of physical exercises and the final one is the headstand; when you have done the headstand, you stand back again on your feet for as long as you have stood on the head, and then you lie down in the corpse posture. The entire practice of hatha yoga as an act of worship, as an act of ritual, is an enactment of the cycle of creation and dissolution, an enactment of the cycle of birth and death. You start with a deep breath, and end with a corpse; you die daily, and thereby you become immortal. The only way to gain immortality is to take a little death serum every day—this is the principle of immunity. So you lie in the corpse posture, you become relaxed, and then that leads to meditation. This is one way of transition from hatha into meditation.

Second is through pranayama. The exercise of the physical body leads to deepening of the breath. Deepening of the breath leads to control of prana, and that leads into meditation.

The third route is through the natural practice of asanas. When your body is totally under your control, your posture comes under control; and when you can keep your body in a certain posture for a long time, the mind struggles, struggles, struggles to move the body, but one part of your will says, "No, I am going to stay like this"— and then the mind stops its fight and becomes still, and is led into meditation. A number of Tibetan monasteries for beginning practice of meditation use that; just sit down over a long period of time and say, "I shall not move." A long period of time does not mean one hour, two hours; it means eight hours, it means three years, three months, three days, three hours of sitting in one place and not even being able to stretch the body fully. So this is the third avenue, stillness of the body, accomplished through the perfection of a posture, which is the hard way, but leads ultimately to the stillness of the mind.

And then the fourth way is through the perfection of the six *kriyas* of hatha yoga explained in all major books on the subject. The final *kriya* is *trataka*. You start with eye exercise, move on to gazing; gazing becomes concentration; and concentration, prolonged, becomes meditation.

4

The Whole Body Language

In the Yoga Sutras of Patanjali there are three aphorisms on posture which we shall study below. The first is Sutra II.46: *Sthira-sukham asanam*, "A posture should be steady and comfortable." The posture should be not only steady, not only comfortable, but steady *and* comfortable. Suffice it to say that when one becomes steady without feeling discomfort, then the asana is perfected. It is not only that one should choose an asana, a posture, which is steady and comfortable, but when one sits in the asana in a steady manner over a long period of time without feeling discomfort, that is the perfection of the asana. One starts with a steady and comfortable posture but then perfects that posture by making it steady without discomfort.

The second sutra we will study is Sutra II.47: *Prayatna-shaithilyananta-samapattibhyam*, "(The posture is perfected, made steady and comfortable) through relaxing (not forcing) the effort and by fixing the consciousness on the infinite." The founder and spiritual guide of the Himalayan Institute, Swami Rama, describes two kinds of asanas: the asanas of physical culture and the asanas of meditation. This sutra is concerned with the asanas of meditation, but to a certain extent, the asanas of physical culture also are meditative asanas and cannot be accomplished without a meditative attitude. There are two versions of the sutra; one reads *ananta-samapattibhyam,* the other reads *anantya-samapattibhyam.* We shall discuss both versions.

On one hand, hatha is called force, but the sooner the force is abandoned and relaxation is used to perfect the asana the better. The effort and the movement should be natural. In taking the other meaning of the word hatha— *ha,* the sun; *tha,* the moon—the breath rhythm employed together with the relaxation of the body and of the mind will help in perfecting the posture. When the mind struggles against the mind and makes the body struggle against the body while doing asanas, it is not the way to perfect a posture. The mind should be completely relaxed and the effort should be a relaxed effort with very natural rhythmic movement—with relaxed limbs and mind. Then the asana will be perfected much more easily and more comfortably.

For this reason, one of the secrets of perfecting an asana is to do it over and over again mentally, as it were almost fantasizing that you are doing the asana. As it was explained in chapter 1, go through each asana in your mind as if you were doing it, and observe the entire mental process. For any asana that will be the first prerequisite.

A teacher of hatha yoga should spend some time with the class doing the asana mentally. In fact, before starting the class with the asana, he or she should describe and demonstrate the asana while the students relax their bodies and minds completely. They should first observe and then visualize themselves going through all the movements. The entire body movement should be grasped, not only the held position, but everything that will lead gracefully to and from the held position. Beginners should mentally experience the easy, natural, beautiful flow of movements that will lead them effectively and gracefully through the asana. Let them do that mentally, meditatively, and then tell them to do with the body what their minds already did. Eventually, in the process of doing the asana mentally, they will recognize the obstacles that are present and will begin to soothe and smooth them out in that mental process. As they smooth them out in the mental process, gradually the physical resistance, which is tension, will be removed and the asana will become steady without discomfort. So that is *prayatna-shaithilya,* relaxing the effort.

The other reading of this sutra is *ananta-samapatti-bhyam,* fixing the mind on infinity, concentration on the infinite. The meaning of the word infinite may be twofold. One meaning has to do with the limited concept we have of our body as a material object occupying such and such a place in time. Observe it this way: the body is heavy; it has a feeling for gravity. This gravitational feeling, heaviness, *guruta,* is responsible for our rigidness. When the mind is taken beyond limitations of time, space, and causation to which the physical body is subject, then the entire personality becomes part of the infinite. What cannot be easily manipulated within the context of these rigidities of time, space, and sequence becomes easily manipulated when it is seen as part of the infinite.

It seems somewhat impossible at this stage that a student who is just beginning to practice yoga can expect his mind to become fixed on the infinite to such an extent that the body will attain perfection of the asana without much effort. It seems that the means, *sadhana,* is becoming the end, *sadhya,* and *sadhya* is becoming *sadhana.* The means seem to become the very goal itself. The purpose of the highest concentration, the highest samadhi, is to have the mind fixed on the infinite, and these asanas and so on are all the means. *Asana,* the third means of the limbs of Ashtanga Yoga, will be perfected by the mind being fixed on the ultimate infinite consciousness. If we take this particular interpretation of the sutra, then the sutra says that if you really reach the ultimate, then all of these limbs are automatically perfected. After all, who taught yoga to Saint Francis of Assisi? Who taught yoga to the first founder of the yoga system? Because their minds were fixed, the asana was perfected without effort.

To digress here for a few pages, there is in theological circles always a controversy as to whether certain miraculous powers, or accomplishments, *siddhis* in Sanskrit, are a gift of grace or whether they are earned by hard work, so to speak. In the tradition of Christianity there is a precept that, for example, the power to heal the sick or the power to cast out devils or the power to speak in tongues are all gifts from the Holy Spirit, and that we do not really earn them. This is a very interesting topic and it is not a problem limited to Christian theology. The question of acts and grace, our preparation and God's gift, is part of practical metaphysics.

The yogi's standard answer is that even when we speak of the *siddhi* being acquired, you first gain the qualification. Why is it that I do not have a certain gift? Why, for example, can't I walk up to a wolf and say, "Look, brother wolf, don't bite people," and have brother wolf say, "All right, Saint, I won't." Why don't I have that power? Why is God so partial that he would give that power to Saint Francis and not to me? The answer, Christian, Hindu, or

Japanese, would be that we receive the gift when we are the right vessels. An ocean cannot be poured into a pint-sized bottle. Our minds have to be expanded through our prayer, longing, self-purification, discipline, and through our concentration. The effort is not toward attaining the *siddhi*, toward getting the gift. The gift is ever present, always here, because God is all-pervading, within reach of everyone. The effort is in purifying ourselves to the extent that we become the right vessels for the gift. I have really no doubt that Swami Rama, called "Swamiji" as a gesture of affection and respect, would say ultimately that the gift (the acquisition of a *siddhi*) comes as a by-product of our efforts toward self-purification. And until that certain level of self-purification is reached, the ever-present gifts are there, but we are not large enough packages to contain them.

This also applies to instantaneous samadhi. Take the question of someone like Saint Paul, who is an archenemy of Christ and then suddenly he finds his eyes closing. A light strikes and for three days he cannot open his eyes. Ordinarily, we train people to close their eyes, but then there are some fortunate people who never have to train themselves to close them. When the light strikes, the eyes are blinded. In the case of Saint Paul, his burst of enmity against Christ was like the last flicker of a candle dying, like the last flicker of the force of negative *samskaras* spending itself out in a quick burst and being done with it. As soon as that vestige was spent, he was ready for the sudden strike of grace, even from a disembodied master. In such cases everything that would happen to a person studying and practicing over a long period of time happens instantaneously. The way the process of evolution seems to work with the human fetus is that in nine months it passes through the stages that life passed through in nine million or ninety million years. You look back and see from where you have come. The same thing happens in the practice of meditation. Everything that one has practiced in the past lives, one starts again in each life right from the beginning. But the level he had reached in ten previous lifetimes he will reach in ten months in this lifetime; and people will say that he is making unusually fast progress and that he is precocious, gifted!

When the soul has reached a certain point, it becomes a *sakadagami bodhisattva,* a potential buddha who will return only once more to perfect himself, or an *anagami bodhisattva,* one who will no longer return to perfect himself except as an incarnate perfected being. Also in such a case he goes through all ascetic practices very quickly and comes to final realization. So also a teacher may see a person who comes to the first day of class and sits down in the lotus posture and goes through the relaxation exercise and says, "I feel whirls, whirls of energy, something burning around me." When a teacher sees such a person, he becomes excited, really excited, because he knows that the student has practiced it all before.

When you are opening yourself to the infinite consciousness, the asana automatically becomes perfected because the infinite is the Absolute. And the steadiness of your personality is the Absoluteness, *kaivalya,* the goal of yoga as defined in the last chapters of the Yoga Sutras. Sometimes a yogi is seen to be so still that you would not think that there was life in him. Our Swamiji becomes so still that you would think the flesh had turned into marble.

So, returning to Sutra II.47, this infinite consciousness as a means in order to perfect an asana does not make sense. It is no help saying that obtaining infinite consciousness will perfect your posture. It is like draining a whole ocean to get one block of ice.

Now, the second interpretation of the sutra is "Concentration on empty space perfects the asana." If you send your mind out to the entire expanse of space, you can imagine and find that very space passing through you. If your mind can go and capture this—it is not the true infinity but what appears like infinity to the mind, that infinity-like nature, extent, expansion of space, that very space being around you, that very space passing through you—it will help you attain lightness of the body without too much effort. In other words the relaxation of effort, the first means shown in the sutra, is helped by concentration on the concept of space. Because, what are you? Your whole framework is made up of perhaps ninety percent space from head to toe. So what is it you are trying to twist when you do the asana? Is it not empty space? What is the problem then when you are trying to twist empty space?

If the nucleus of a hydrogen atom were the size of an apple, then the electron would be forty feet away. The scientists are thrilled by the discovery of a new subatomic particle, the psi particle. This particle lasts for one hundred millionth of a millionth of a second. That is its lifespan. It shows how fine a time-division of a material particle they are capable of capturing. If an atomic particle is capable of capturing that, the human mind, the finest form of material energy, is capable in meditation of concentrating on a microscopic division of time that is finer still. We should understand this concept of space and its relationship to physical bodies, and know that this body is for the most part nothing but empty space. What then is it that is giving us so much trouble in twisting? If we could get the feel of this idea, the experience of it, then we would have no problem mastering an asana.

A third interpretation of the sutra is somewhat mythological, a philosophical interpretation couched in mythical language. Mythology is nothing but philosophy given an interesting symbolic form. Philosophy taken to the subconscious mind becomes mythology. All the figures arise from there. It can be a *sattvic, rajasic,* or *tamasic* form. Philosophy at the heart level, at the emotional level, is mythology. So the sutra is given a mythological interpretation in which the word *ananta* is the name of the great snake on whom the Lord Vishnu sleeps. *Ananta* means "non-ending, eternal, infinite." Its other name is *Shesha,* which means "the residue." When the universe is dissolved, Vishnu, God the Preserver, sleeps on the coiled-up snake of infinity that is the residue, the remainder, of the universe. It is said in the mythological tradition that this earth is supported on the million heads of Ananta, this snake. And the snake is in turn supported by a turtle. The attainment of the *siddhi* of asanas is the satisfaction of that turtle. When the turtle moves, the snake moves, and when the snake moves, the whole earth shakes.

In the yoga language, stripping the beautiful imagery, we know the snake to be the kundalini. When the kundalini becomes firm, not shaking, the whole body becomes firm, becomes like a flame in a place where there is no breeze, no wind. Everything becomes steady—voice, eyes, hearing, senses, words, mind, posture, standing, sitting—everything.

When a yogi sees a person who cannot be steady he feels very unhappy, very sorry. We may move about freely out of choice; we can dance, or just stand relaxed, but we should be consciously aware of it. At a moment's notice we should be able to be still; there should be no more movement in us. Our mind should become fixed on one point, and there should be no movement from that point. As long as we wish, we should remain concentrated on that one point. Then we would have conquest of emotion. A person who moves and shakes about uncontrollably is emotionally disturbed. A person who has steady emotion has a settled, calm body and a steady voice. The perfection of a posture has all these ramifications. It is not merely that we can put our body into such-and-such a position. What is our posture like when we are walking, standing, or talking at a party? Drama schools train actresses to maintain good posture. That becomes artificial because it does not come from the steadiness of emotions and of mind. When a person cannot be steady and has to speak, speak, speak, eat, eat, eat, move, move, move, there is something emotionally disturbed there.

The first thing we have to do is straighten our lives. If the mind is divided four ways, the posture will be divided four ways. That is where the whole body language comes in. The more we grow, the more we should become aware of our posture. Let the emotions work on the posture and at the same time let the posture train the emotions.

At a weekend retreat some years ago a lot of people began to complain of having to sit still for fifteen minutes without moving. If a person cannot sit firm for fifteen minutes he will probably quit a job in fifteen days, or will not stay in a college course for fifteen days. Nor will he remain loyal to the same wife for fifteen years, because the emotional steadiness is missing. He will run, run, run and try to escape all the time. The perfection of posture shows itself generally in daily life; walking, working in a hospital, sitting behind a typewriter, show something about a person. When someone has that perfection of posture, then his words come out differently. So many people talk or speak from the front of the mouth because nothing is coming from the depth of the heart or from the depth of the mind. The whole body posture is slack and the words coming out are slack. There is no point, no direction to them, they are not channeled. The mind is not channeled.

In Indian mythology Vishnu, the sustaining, nurturing aspect of God, who pervades the whole universe-body and our personal bodies, upon the dissolution of the universe, rests on the coiled-up snake of kundalini. The perfection of the spine is the perfection of the postures because the spine is the seat of the kundalini. That is why when a teacher is teaching someone to perfect the lotus posture, he advises the student to shift his legs but to keep the spine straight. We need to have an axis, the *meru,* which is the central mountain of the earth in yoga symbolism, on one side of which the sun rises, on the other side of which the sun sets. One of the Sanskrit words for the spine is *meru-danda,* the meru pole (meridian). The spine is *meru-danda,* the axis pole of the body, and if our axis line is straight then the rest of the body is well balanced.

The snake Shesha or Ananta rests on the back of the turtle. What is the turtle? There is a passage from the Bhagavad Gita and also from St. Teresa of Avila that says: "As a turtle draws in his limbs, so a man of wisdom withdraws all his senses." That is the turtle. Another yoga sutra of Patanjali (III.31) is: *Kurma-nadyam sthairyam:* by concentration on the *kurma-nadi,* the turtle channel of prana in the vicinity of the cardiac center, one attains the *siddhi* of *sthairya,* perfection of steadiness and stillness. When you have withdrawn your senses the way a turtle draws in his limbs, only then the snake of infinity in you can rest straight and support all the pervading life force in you on its thousand heads. When the turtle shakes, the snake moves and the earth quakes. The posture changes.

The power of the kundalini is such that it not only moves everything, it stills everything, because the impulses of the kundalini are finer than any particle of matter discovered; as a result your mind when concentrated becomes so finely tuned to one single point in time, space, and sequence that you enter and stay there. The whole body becomes firm. All you have to do is to find that point. So by concentrating on this snake of infinite space the posture is corrected and perfected. Think of a snake which has been stretched out and straightened, and that is your spine.

We have given here several different methods of perfecting one's posture. The perfection of the posture, remember, should not be perfection of the yoga postures at the time of doing hatha. It is the perfection of a posture throughout life. And that is an indication of where one's mind is. A person may relax, bend the spine, stand any way he wants. That is all right, but his command of himself should be such that instantaneously and for any length of time he could keep his spine straight, use that as an axis and let his mind move gracefully. If we know about the snake, no one has to teach us to dance after that. The more steadiness we have in our minds, the more grace we will derive from there, and the more controlled and graceful our movement will become.

A person should work on the condition of the mind that disturbs his posture. Then the posture itself will automatically correct itself and will perfect itself. What is it in the mind that makes a person move? Whatever it is in the mind that makes him move from his physical posture is the same thing that makes him escape from a relational situation, that prevents him from sticking to any subject over a long period of time, that causes him to marry once and then marry again and then marry a third time, that makes him teacher-hop and mantra-shop; that makes him hop here and shop there. That is the rabbit posture!

The third sutra we will study is Sutra II.48: *Tato dvandvanabhighatah,* "Then one no (longer) suffers from pairs of opposites (such as heat and cold)." Then one is not troubled, disturbed, by the *dvandvas;* not getting hurt, not suffering, not being perturbed, by the *dvandvas.* The word *dvandva* means pairs of opposites, dichotomies. There are all kinds of pairs of opposites in this world. The entire world consists of two. When two becomes one, the world ceases. If space, time, causation, all become one and there is no past versus future, no here versus there, then the two have become one. Similarly, if we have two choices, a conflict, an emotional two-ness, a double-mindedness, we have a split within ourselves, a schizophrenia, because there is this preoccupation with two simultaneously. Our minds are split. An emotional duality, spiritual duality, physical duality, develops, and we are entangled in the pairs of opposites—heat versus cold, pain versus pleasure, and so on.

Thus we human beings even cast our heaven in the images of our own minds, so that the mythology that developed around Mesopotamia, Arabia, and Israel, in the deserts and hot parts of the world, always depicts hell as burning hot. The hell of the Middle Eastern mythology is all fire, whereas the Middle Eastern heavens were imagined as cool places under the shade of vines with grapes hanging from them that you do not have to reach for, they just fall into your mouth. In the Koran, you will find heaven is depicted there with canals of cool water flowing, because the only happiness and pleasure people found in Arabia was in the shade of an oasis. But the hell of Nordic mythology is a very dark cold place, all ice. Whatever we long for in this life but do not get, we hope to get in the next life. There is always a wish, a hope, and that longing becomes our heaven. But in reality there is neither heaven nor hell, but only the pairs of opposites playing on our minds.

When a person has perfected his meditative asana he is no longer perturbed by the pairs of opposites. When the axis of the spine is straight and firm and neither falls to the left nor the right, nor front nor backwards, there is perfect balance. Both the centrifugal and centripetal forces are so well balanced that they do not let the whirling top fall, because the axis is there. When you have found your axis in life, it shows itself in your posture. You stand firm with your body, with your emotions, and then you are not easily distracted by heat and cold, or pain and pleasure, or craving and satisfaction, or praise and blame. You watch the *dvandvas* with dispassion as a witness, and that becomes your natural discipline.

When disciples are trained in the caves of the Himalayas, the masters do not simply begin by teaching them the Yoga Sutras on the first day, but they make them sit. Everybody wants to go to the caves of the Himalayas, but many people cannot sit still for six minutes in meditation, let alone six hours. What is needed is the conquest of that pain, conquest of the principle of opposites. But if we just force our bodies to withstand the pain, we will not succeed. It is the duality of the mind between pain and pleasure that has to be conquered, that has to be unified.

So conquest of the pairs of opposites is a natural result of the perfection of posture. But if you do not conquer it in your daily emotional life and are torn all the time between *this* and *that,* then you cannot sit long for meditation, because the mind controls and moves the axis of the body. The mind is shifting all the time, all twenty-four hours. The mind is shifting during meditation, shifting the axis, tilting the axis and the *meru-danda.* The central mountain begins to quake, so you have earthquakes in the body, and it twitches and has spasms.

Here is the true meaning of asceticism. The true meaning of asceticism is not to withstand the heat and cold and go catch a cold by walking on snow, but to become such a person that you walk in snow in ordinary cottons without catching a cold. Find in the mind where the posture begins, and from there send the right impulse, the right direction, and that is then the perfection of the posture. That way you are no longer subjected to the vagaries of extreme cravings. In the city of Kanpur I heard that for seven days our Swamiji sat with no food, no water, no movement, no toilet, no bath. He just sat for seven days, at one spot.

Posture is the firmness of mind, firmness of emotions, firmness of life, firmness of decision. It is a whole body language.

5

Kundalini—
The Coiled-Up Energy

We have spoken of hatha yoga as worship, as asceticism, and as a means of purifying karma. Now let us briefly discuss it in relation to kundalini yoga. Kundalini yoga is the yoga of energy currents, not in the sense of electric energy or heat energy or light energy, which are material, but in the sense of *living* energy, which is I, the Self, "That I Am." The mainstream of the kundalini flows through the spine divided into three streams, *ida, pingala,* and *sushumna: sushumna,* the mainstream; *ida* to the left; *pingala* to the right. When *pingala* is active, the right nostril flows freely; when *ida* is active, the left nostril flows freely.

In kundalini yoga, the coiled-up energy lying in the lower center of consciousness is awakened. Only a very minor portion, a very minor current, of the kundalini is awake in most of us and keeps us going through the totality of all the experiences and activities of our lives. All the functions of consciousness—the brain, the senses, movements, nerves, desires, passions, complexes—everything that we are or do, everything that we are aware of— thought and action processes, experiences, memories,

71

inventions, genius, poetry, sex, violence and murder, peace and quietude and tranquility—are functions of the kundalini force. A minute amount is released into our system through the spine, connecting to the brain and to the seven centers of consciousness. From there it is distributed through the entire system: the warmth in our hands, the light in our eyes, the taste in our mouths, the speech on our tongues, and so on. Everything that mankind has acquired, attained, developed, evolved, achieved, created, destroyed, is a minute spark of kundalini. This energy is not only *sat,* existence as in matter, but also *chit,* consciousness, awareness, life, a ray of God, brilliant like ten thousand suns, a streak of lightning in the spine.

A yogi's ultimate aim is the total awakening of kundalini and when that awakening takes place, the yogi's consciousness thereafter is the entire life force which exists in the whole universe. The yogi realizes that he is plugged into it and walks in that consciousness. It is from this that all the miraculous powers are derived by the yogi. He lives in an entirely different world, and yet he appears to be doing nothing unusual, for he does not need to move his body to do kundalini yoga. Kundalini yoga is a very high and very subtle form of yoga in which nothing happens that is visible to others. It is the yoga of real intangibles, to which maybe one out of five hundred million humans may have access.

Hatha yoga in its finest, highest, deepest philosophy is a preparation for kundalini yoga. Hatha yoga is, then, the preparation for the control and direction of meditative experience. In very simple terms, we know we have a problem sitting to meditate. Once we have solved the problem of feet falling asleep, then other problems really begin, because from that point on we become more and more aware of what a hindrance this gross body and its gross habits are to the experience of anything finer. Hatha yoga is refining the body to move a human being to a finer energy existence.

How many angels dance on a pinhead? Five, fifty, five hundred? How can so many angels dance on a pinhead? Because they are not made of gross matter but are beings of energy. In meditation we become aware of this. The ultimate aim of yoga is the total transformation of humanity into beings of pure divine energy. Arthur C. Clarke's *Childhood's End* comes very close to the aspiration that human beings have had for a long time to become angelic, to become beings of energy, like *devas* (the shining ones), so that they do not need a gross physical body. What we experience of the sensuous, sensual world with our senses is only a very minute portion of the experiences that truly exist on the level of energy. In kundalini yoga, those experiences of a finer world unfold. Initially, the experiences of kundalini are very pleasant, so pleasant that the physical or sensual experiences that people are familiar with become as nothing compared to the kundalini sensations. Even though a yogi may use sense experiences for intangible internal purposes of which few people have any understanding, he does not identify with them or derive the pleasure from them that we do.

A person may come to a hatha yoga class to learn about how to strengthen his back. Such things as strengthening the back and working on thyroid problems are very easy, but hatha yoga as a preparation for higher steps of meditation is something else. As I said before, we start from a very gross level. If the spine is not straight, the energy flow is obstructed. Hatha yoga is the cranking of a motorcar engine: the inside switch is not working, so you go out and crank the engine, using force. However, when you know how the spark plugs operate, how the ignition works, then you work from within. Kundalini yoga is working from within, whereas hatha yoga is working from the outside.

Let us take just this very basic fact of knowledge of kundalini yoga: that *sushumna* is an energy stream flowing through the spine, passing through seven centers of consciousness as if it were a river with seven lakes on its way. This river is called Sarasvati (*saras* means a lake). Unless a person has learned how to keep his spine straight, he will block that energy flow where it goes out into finer currents, into the capillaries, into millions of nerve endings, and so forth. The power of that energy flow depends on how straight the spine is. If the spine and neck are not straight, then the rib cage will not be lifted up properly. The kundalini energy will then not be stimulated well by the deep flow of the breath, nor will the breath be stimulated well by the smooth flow of the kundalini energy.

There are four locks, or *bandhas*, practiced in hatha yoga: *mulabandha*, the root lock, which is the pulling up of the lower anal-genital sphincter muscles and internal rectal muscles; *khechari*, the tongue lock, which is turning the tongue up and back into the palate as far back as it will go; *uddiyana bandha*, pulling in the stomach, creating a hole as you pull in and up into the rib cage; and *jalandhara bandha*, locking the throat, pushing the chin into the hollow between the collarbones. A fifth lock, *jnana-mudra* or *chin-mudra*, locking the fingers for meditation, is easily achieved by gently touching the tips of the index fingers to the tips of the thumbs so that the energy flow is not going outward but is drawn back around inward and locked. The fingers naturally assume this comfortable position and curve together like those of a baby.

When *mulabandha,* the anal lock, is accomplished, the next step is the practice of *ashvini mudra. Ashvini mudra* is a release and pulling of the root lock. Leave the rest of the body relaxed and pull the anal lock up and in, and release . . . and pull . . . and release . . . and pull . . . and release. It pulls in the entire area. If Roman Catholic priests were taught some of these exercises, the practice of celibacy would become easier for them, because they would be able to take the downward-outward flowing energy and pull it upward and inward, from lower centers (*chakras*) of consciousness relating to sexual thoughts to higher centers where feelings of love and compassion predominate, such as the *anahata chakra,* the heart center. The idea in kundalini yoga is to raise energy up into higher centers of consciousness. As you raise the energy into these higher centers, you are able to accomplish much more from each center than you could accomplish before. When the heart center is opened, for example, it is not that you become unemotional but rather that you become a master of your own emotions and of those emotions to which you are exposed around you. Or, when the throat center is open, you become a master of music and song as well as of hunger and thirst. When the center between the eyebrows is opened, you become master of all insights and intuitive processes.

In kundalini yoga, nothing is seen happening. A yogi may be sitting before your very eyes; you do not see anything happening because he is not moving his physical body in any specific way. But what moves is the finer energy current within. Hatha yoga becomes a preparation for the inner movement. When one is, let us say, pulling in and releasing the anal lock, the idea is not just moving the muscles. Most people move the muscles in and out and that accomplishes very little. When you perform the *ashvini mudra,* releasing and holding, releasing and holding, the current should be felt all the way up to the seventh center.

> Sit with your head, neck and trunk straight. Close your eyes. Relax your mind. Relax your forehead. Relax your facial muscles. Relax your jaw.
>
> Relax your jaw more. Relax your shoulders. Relax the shoulders until you feel the relaxation in the fingertips. Relax your chest and your rib cage. Relax your cardiac center.
>
> Relax your stomach, navel, abdomen. Relax your pelvis, and all the muscles of your legs.
>
> Relax your legs again. Relax your pelvis. Relax the base of your spine. Bring your attention to the groups of vertebrae in your spine. Pay attention to your vertebrae and relax your vertebrae one by one. (You will not be able to do this unless your posture is correct.)
>
> Relax your shoulder blades. Relax your shoulders. Relax your jaw. Relax your face and forehead. Exhale and inhale, feeling the breath in your nostrils—as if the breath begins from the center between the eyebrows.
>
> Now, as you breathe in, feel as if the breath is going down your spine, all the way down to the base of the spine. As you exhale, feel as if the breath is flowing up the spinal column; inhale without a pause, as if the breath is going in and down into the very base of the spine. As the breath flows up and out, it is as if the energy current is flowing upward.
>
> Breathing in, down the spine, repeat your mantra. Breathing out, up the spine, think your mantra.
>
> Keep your cardiac center relaxed. Keep your shoulders relaxed. Keep your jaw and forehead relaxed. Keep your spine straight. Breathing in, think the mantra. Breathing out, think the mantra in the spine.

Now as you breathe up the spine, pull your rectal, anal-sphincter muscles upward as if you were pushing all the energies into the spinal flow from the lower centers upward. As you inhale, the breath flows downward with the mantra, and as you flow upward through the spine, push the energy with the root lock as if that push is felt all the way up through the breath. Be aware only of that flow.

There is a tendency to release this energy and tension in the mouth, so turn your tongue up and back into the palate; create a suction in your cheeks and the sides of your jaw. Relax your shoulders. Relax your cardiac center. Continue to feel the inhalation down the spine. Exhale up the spine with the tongue lock and the root lock. When you exhale, feel as if the root lock is pushing up the energy into your spine.

Let there be no tension on your face. Maintain the mantra with each breath. Continue to feel this flow while slowly opening your eyes.

Here you have a combination of hatha yoga (doing something with your muscles), mantra yoga (observing the mantra in the mind), and kundalini yoga (concentrating on the kundalini flow).

What we do in hatha yoga by force and will power happens naturally and involuntarily later when the kundalini awakens. Let us look at the inner washes in yoga. The inner washes are excellent practices to undertake in order to maintain good health. They accomplish their purpose by freeing the body of all built-up poisons and cleansing the lymph nodes, digestive system, and all the rest. When a yogi practicing kundalini yoga is using those washes, he has another purpose at the same time. If there are particles of food in the system when sitting down to meditate, a yogi becomes aware of them, so he has to keep his insides clean. Furthermore, the cleansing that is accomplished voluntarily in hatha yoga washes—taking in water and expelling it, for example—begins to happen automatically in kundalini yoga. It is much like the involuntary cleansing a woman experiences a short time before menstruation. Once every month, or even more often, the yogi might have a diarrhea-like experience with all waste matter being forcibly expelled because of the kundalini energy acting on the vagus nerve. As the vagus nerve is stimulated, it has effects not only on the thinking and brain energy but also on the entire autonomic nervous system. There is scientific evidence that if the vagus nerve were stimulated electrically, for example, there would be a similar type of situation. No one, however, has learned how to do that voluntarily yet except the kundalini yogis, who stimulate the vagus nerve that way through the central energy channel in the spine known as *sushumna.*

When one becomes aware of the kundalini currents, he also becomes aware of many things in the body that an average person does not notice. He knows exactly what the state of his stomach is, what the state of his lungs is, what his liver is doing, and how his brain is functioning; he knows at all times how his breath is flowing. By breathing a certain way he can lie down, perhaps begin dictating a book, and condense three hours of sleep into one hour. When the physical breath becomes connected to the prana force which is connected to the kundalini breath, the yogi generates so much energy that he can get a full night's rest in a short time using a special technique called *yoga nidra* (yoga sleep).

There are other exercises in hatha yoga which are meant primarily for the awakening of kundalini. For example, the *mahamudra* is a simple practice of pushing the heel against the perineum and stretching out one leg, keeping the sole of the other foot parallel to the thigh, holding the toe of the stretched-out foot, and pulling oneself forward or backward. This exerts a pressure on an area known as the *yoni-kanda* which is the *svadhishthana,* the seat of the Mother, the kundalini. As the root lock is established and you try to pull your toe, the pressure is increased even more. With the awareness of breath, a certain concentration is felt in the lower centers. If you do not know the art, the concentration of energies in the lower centers can mislead you. If you know the art and are initiated by a master, you are taught how to take that energy and lead it up into the higher centers of consciousness. One of the best times to meditate is when there is a strong sexual desire. Then that crypto-sexual energy goes upward and you have the deepest possible meditations.

Many students are puzzled about what place sexual activity has in yoga. The subject of the relationship of kundalini and sexual energy is a very complex one. A forced celibacy is of no use. What is celibacy? Celibacy is the senses being fully potent yet not desirous of their objects. Celibacy is not an abstinence from indulging the senses; celibacy is the senses not being inclined to the indulgence. Celibacy, then, is of the mind, not of the body. The subject is only for the initiate, for someone who has gone through the experiences of the kundalini. The first recommendation to the seeker is to be natural and normal regarding sexual activity but not to be overindulgent; to try to limit sexual relations to once a week for those who have an established partner. But even more important is that when one is engaging in sex, let the indulgence be limited to that time alone and not to other times. That is celibacy. For a normal, Western man who is not a Catholic

priest and who is not aiming at becoming a monk or a
renunciate, the recommendation is that when you are
eating, enjoy the food at that time and do not crave it at
other times. That is true celibacy. It is not that a person
refuses to speak when his tongue itches to talk, but that the
tongue no longer wishes to speak. And when the person
does speak, it is no more than is absolutely necessary, and
it is beneficial and pleasant to people. That is celibacy.
Celibacy is mind not craving too much.

"Why not?" people ask. "Why not indulge the senses?
The senses are beautiful." Indeed, they are beautiful—but
because your diamonds are beautiful, you do not throw
them around out in the street every day. You safeguard
them and protect them. A person who aspires for meditative progress must fully understand that the outward,
downward scattering of energy that goes out in one's
overindulgence of the senses, uncontrolled movement of
the body, uncontrolled movement of the eyes, ears,
stomach, sex, heart, emotion, speech, or whatever else, is
taking away from an inward, upward flow of energy. That
is the only connection between celibacy and spirituality.
Senses are not sinful. This is where the puritanical attitude
of the Western idea of celibacy differs from the yoga
tradition. In yoga the attempt is to bring the senses to their
fullest power and yet learn to divert their direction to an
inward, upward flow.

What we need to practice is celibacy of the mind.
Celibacy of an emotion is not suppression of a desire, but
non-inclination. How do we do that? Only by replacing a
lower desire with a higher, sublime one. If we just try to
suppress a sexual desire, it's not healthy. It will come out
in one way or another. But if I know that this very energy
can make my meditation blossom and I have a desire for

meditation, after a period of time a natural inclination toward meditation will develop.

What are blocks in the *chakras*? On what level do they occur? Until the flowers of our consciousness—one, two, three, four, five, six, seven flowers of consciousness—are in full bloom, they are all blocked. Because the heart center is blocked, there are warps in our emotions; there is inability to love all universally because the heart is blocked. Because the navel center is blocked, there are all sorts of cravings. Because the sexual center is blocked, there is a downward, outward flow of sexual energy instead of an inward, upward flow. Because the throat center is blocked, my words will not reverberate around this planet for two thousand years the way the Sermon on the Mount has reverberated.

Removal of those blocks is a long and gradual process. Sometimes it may be a very dramatic experience, but in most cases it is gradual and slow. Something begins to happen, but you cannot be working in four different directions at once. There are people who claim to be followers of kundalini yoga and say "Love everybody" and "Have sex with everybody." The two statements are contradictory. To love everybody means opening of the heart center—an upward, inward flow. Having sex with everybody is blocking the lower center, the sexual center of consciousness, so that the kundalini energy flows downward and outward and is dissipated. When it flows inward and upward, the heart center receives that energy and opens up its love to everyone.

Unless one understands these higher purposes in hatha yoga, hatha yoga remains only a fine physical body exercise. Ultimately, however, hatha yoga is a preparation for the body to contain the kundalini with the establishment of the locks. When the energy force rises, it tries to move you. Some people begin to sway to and fro, left and right; some sweat; some may even shake involuntarily. Kundalini yoga, however, is a highly controlled experience beyond anybody's imagination, something in which the body is absolutely still. The higher you go, the more your body, your emotions, and your brain waves all go still. And the intensity of the field is such that you have to know how to keep that intensity, keep its strength without moving, without shaking.

The locks and postures prepare the body for things that will happen when you begin to become a being of energy, when you begin to realize not that you have a subtle body but that you are the subtle being; that this being has come and permeated and pervaded the physical shape. You realize that a being of energy has come and taken possession of a statue, an image made of plastic, and made it come alive, and that when you touch this plastic statue you are not touching the living being. The living being is pure energy. Kundalini yoga is the yoga of what this energy being does with him*self*, not what he/she/it does with this body. Hatha yoga is what is done with this body to lead toward that realization of being this energy being.

As these preparations begin—gradually in the physical body as well as in the breath and the little fine currents and awareness in the spine or the nosebridge center—people begin to experience a little sensation. What a yogi can accomplish with the force of his kundalini is unthinkable. He is a being of energy. Energy has no weight; it occupies no space; it is invisible. What is happening there is intangible. If you see an electric live wire not covered by any insulation, can you say whether it is alive or not just by looking at it? You cannot. Yet what is happening there is intensely dynamic, intensely active. That is kundalini yoga. The body in hatha yoga moves; the body in kundalini yoga is intensively active but does not move. Who is active? Not the body but the being of energy which has come and taken possession of this lifelong statue.

If one goes into the practice of meditation and has not trained the body, then one's practice of meditation is delayed. One needs to learn to sit crosslegged, crossing the hands in the lap in the lotus posture or joining the fingers, closing the energy circles, pulling in the root lock, the anal lock, pulling in the tongue, gathering all the energies in and making a nice, neat bundle. Now it is an internally active dynamo. No energy is being passed out but the prana is being activated. Breathe out, breathe in, breathe out, breathe in. The dynamo is creating energy within itself. It is being activated and intensified constantly without the loss of energy through the eyes or through the tongue or through the sexual apparatus or through anywhere else. Through intense concentration, the awareness is brought to one single point so that the energy that is lost through the awareness of various objects is pulled in and made, again, into a laser beam.

When you perform your hatha yoga, do it with the awareness of these energies. Do not merely move muscles when doing hatha yoga. The muscles move anyway, but the purpose is to locate the field of energy.

We have referred to the philosophy of posture according to Patanjali, which is finding your axis, *axis mundi,* axis of the world. It is this area known as *meru-danda,* from the base of the spine to the top of the head. Meru, the central mountain of the universe, on one side of which is

East and on the other side of which is West, that is your axis. Your asana, the sitting posture experience, should be an experience not of holding your hands, legs, and feet in a particular position, but of drawing yourself into this axis. A lot of times, people sit down to meditate and then they try to train their legs. There's a little imbalance, a feeling of a pull toward the right or toward the left. One keeps trying to straighten up but cannot because the legs have not been balanced. When the legs are properly balanced, then the axis is straight. What are legs? Take any ordinary pole that is braced by legs. The legs are supporting and keeping it straight. If the legs are fixed on the ground in a properly balanced manner, the pole will be straight. Pull one of the legs, and it topples over. I know the case of a man who said, "I think I'll sit and practice in a chair." After a while, he said, "I can't; I'm uncomfortable; something happens in meditation, my legs want to pull in." He got into hatha yoga and started training his legs. If in the practice of physical yoga you work from the axis with the awareness of the spine, then you have complete control of the breath and the rest of the energizing apparatus.

A practitioner of hatha yoga should undertake his practice with the aspiration of making his body a fit temple for God—not merely figuratively but literally—to make it a proper vessel for the awakened divine ray called the kundalini. Otherwise, when the spiritual energy begins to build up, the body will be unable to contain it because it has not been trained. Hatha yoga is practiced in order to train the body to serve as a fit vessel for the spirit of God within, so that when the coils of divine energy are uncoiled, the body will not become a hindrance but will be physically ready to receive, channel, and use beneficially the spiritual energy realized and released from within itself.

6

Hatha Yoga: Gateway to the Subtle Body

Sanskrit Maxims (Sutras) Composed by the Author

ओ३म्।।

शक्ति-नाडी-प्रपञ्च इत्येतावान् पुरुषः।।१।।

सर्वं स्थूल-शारीरं व्यष्टि-समष्टि-पुरुषे शक्ति-सूक्ष्म-प्रवाहेभ्य
 आविर्भूय तदाकृतिमेव लभते।।२।।

स्थूल-देह-प्रवृत्तयः सूक्ष्म-प्रवाह-प्रवृत्ति- व्यञ्जिकाः।।३।।

किञ्चिद्-व्यञ्जिका एव।।४।।

हठाच्छक्तिचालनं मृदूनां विशेषम्।।५।।

अन्तः प्रवृत्तेः स्थूल-प्रवृत्तिर्मध्याधिमात्राणाम्।।६।।

शारीरस्सहायो मृदूनां सूक्ष्मो मुख्यो ऽधिमात्राणाम्।।७।।

सहायाभावो मुख्यं विलम्बयेत्।।८।।

तत्र मुख्यं सहायं नियोजयेत्।।९।।

पूर्वं सहायानुयोग आशुकारी सर्वेषाम्।।१०।।

ततः सूक्ष्मे प्रवेशः।।११।।

इति श्री सिद्धयोगिराज रामस्वामिपादशिष्योषर्बुधाचार्य प्रणीतं
 हठकुण्डलिनीसूत्रम्।।

Maxims—Translation of the Above Sūtras

1. Man is a field of energy currents flowing along definite channels.

2. All that is gross and physical (in the macrocosmos and man) is projected from and shaped by the pattern of the subtler essences and currents.

3. All that happens in the physical body is a manifestation of changes in the subtle body and in the energy channels.

4. Only a part of what happens in the subtle body and in the energy channels is manifested on the physical plane.

5. Controls established over the physical body serve as triggers to the states of the subtle body and the energy channels. The slow ones (*mṛdu*) especially need to establish the controls.

6. The changes in the subtle body and the energy channels induce changes on the physical plane.

7. The former (changes in the subtle body) are primary, the latter (changes on the physical plane) auxiliary preparations.

8. The absence of the auxiliary preparations delays progress in the primary ones.

9. The primary ones then force the auxiliary.

10. The prior preparation of the auxiliary prevents delay.

11. Then an entry into the subtle body is gained.

Introduction to Maxims

One often hears yoga teachers speak of a technique as a *rahasya*, a secret among the yogis. It is required that such *rahasyas* be guarded as secretly as possible (*gopanīyaṁ prayatnata-*) and be given only to the qualified initiate, an *adhikārin.* Many who are yet outsiders to the path object strongly and say that it is unfair and wrong to keep truth a secret. They fail to understand that even if a technique or a truth is communicated in words to those who lack insight and capacity for an inner experience, it would still remain a secret, hidden from *their* understanding until verified by practice and experience, and that a technique practiced before its prerequisites are mastered can be harmful.

The more sublime aspects of hatha yoga and associated physical controls are just such secret *rahasyas.* It is a mistake to think of hatha yoga merely as a system of physical exercises. The physical asanas are just a beginning to equip the *sādhaka* for higher experience. This is what hatha yoga is: cleansing, trimming, preparing the equipment—that is, the gross body—so that finally a gateway to the subtle body may be opened with the tools that have been prepared.

Explanation of Maxims

To fully understand the sublime aims of hatha yoga it is first essential to grasp the basic premise of kundalini yoga as stated in maxim 1: Man is a field of energy currents flowing along definite channels. The maxim should be explained by an analogy in the terms of basic physics. If you cover a magnet with a sheet of conductive material and then sprinkle some iron filings on it, what happens? The iron filings arrange themselves in the order of, or along, the magnetic force lines. Only someone totally naive will say that the magnetic currents are flowing along the lines on which the iron filings line up. The more accurate statement will be that the iron filings have arranged themselves according to the pattern of magnetic forces. This is true of the whole universe, and of man. The flotsam and jetsam of the gross, the material dross, though more tangible, has no direction of its own; the direction comes from the invisible currents and undercurrents which lend a form to the gross substances. Man, then, is not essentially a physical configuration; not in kundalini yoga. Man is a pattern of energy channels, *shakti-nāḍīs,* along which his gross body has arranged itself like the iron filings along the magnetic force lines, like straw floating on currents, eddies, whirlpools.

All that is gross and physical (in the macrocosmos and in man) is projected from and shaped by the pattern of the subtler essences and currents. All that happens in the physical body is a manifestation of changes in the subtle body and in the energy channels. Only a part of what happens in the subtle body and in the energy channels is manifested on the physical plane.

Let us study an example for maxims 2-4. Man has an insignificant-looking organ called the navel. It seems to serve no purpose whatsoever once the umbilical cord has been severed in a baby. It is an almost laughable organ, as our association with the terms belly-button and navel-gazing would seem to signify. Yet the word *navel* also connotes the idea of a hub, a nave, the center of a wheel, a *chakra.* Why? It is the visible mark of the solar plexus. The Sanskrit word *nābhi,* from the root *nah,* means the place of tying down, binding. It is not only because of the umbilical cord but also because it is *the* center in which all the cords of energy are tied. It is from this center that 72,000 (350,000 according to some texts, e.g., *Shiva-saṁhitā* II.13) *shakti-nāḍīs,* energy currents, flow out to the rest of the circuitry that is man. No wonder that it is here a new personality, that of the baby's, is tied to the mother's circuitry. Some day, hopefully, Western science will discover that a lot more than physical nourishment passes from the mother into the fetus along this path. In other words, (*a*) (Re maxim 3): The umbilical cord is only a physical manifestation of the navel as the hub of the 72,000 invisible energy channels; (*b*) (Re maxim 4): Only a few of the significant functions arising from this hub are indicated through the physical presence and function of the umbilical cord.

Similar examples can be given to explain many other physiological and psychological phenomena of the body and the gross mind. For example, the Freudian interpretations of the oral-genital complex cannot be understood without realizing the deeper connections and controls of the *shankhinī, vajrinī,* and *kuhū nāḍīs,* the energy channels situated in and flowing between the anal-genital and the oral regions.

A gross mistake is committed by many yoga teachers who try to explain the locations and functions of *chakras* and *shakti-nāḍīs* (especially the major ones—*iḍā, pingalā,* and *sushumnā*). The co-incidence of the *chakras* and *shakti-nāḍīs* with the plexuses and nerves is merely indicative of maxims 3 and 4. Their true significance is beyond.

Works like Rele's *Mysterious Kundalini* have done great service to the proponents of yoga by indicating the coincidence and correlation of the *nāḍīs* and *chakras* with nerves and plexuses. But it would be misleading to assume that the words *shakti-nāḍī* and *chakra* are synonymous respectively with "nerve" and "plexus." "Nerve" and "plexus" are terms limited to the realms of physiology and gross psychology. The significance of *nāḍīs* and *chakras* is far greater, as they are (*a*) flows, patterns, and hub-centers in the circuitry of the subtle body; (*b*) connections and

channels for the flow of forces from the causal body; and
(*c*) above all, energy currents and concentrations of the
universal forces—*prana* (the vital force), *chit* (the consciousness force), and *jīva* (the life force)—flowing along
the microcosmic circuitry which directs the vibrations of
the personality of man. [In trying to interpret the ancient
yoga science to westernised man, let us not sacrifice the
yoga terminology and its deeper definitions. We should
not try to place inaccurate limits on our definitions. The
nāḍīs and *chakras* are far more than nerves and plexuses;
since there are no accurate Western terms available for
nāḍī and *chakra*, let us not try to translate them, just as we
use the word *yoga* untranslated.]

Controls established over the physical body serve as
triggers to the state of the subtle body and the energy
channels. The slow ones (*mṛdu*) especially need to establish the controls. In Patanjali's system (*Yogasūtras* I.21,
22) there are *sādhakas* of varying swiftness of accom-
plishment: *mṛdu*, the slow ones; *madhya*, the average,
middling ones, and *adhimātra*, the swift, intense ones. The
degree of swiftness depends on the strength of their
saṁskāras. Depending on how fast one is bound to the
gross externalized consciousness, the speed of interiorization varies. As a man fallen in the mud cannot hope to
put his hand on a marble floor in order to get up, so a slow
one, *mṛdu sādhaka*, cannot go directly from the gross to
the subtle without first learning to master the physical. The
path from the physical to the subtle body is an intricate one
and only a few fortunate rare ones can find it right at the
beginning of their *sādhana*. The practice of hatha yoga is
absolutely essential for the slow ones. Gradually one learns
to identify the subtler forces and as the controls are
established, the barriers begin to crumble ever so slowly.

At this stage, if the *sādhaka* has guidance on the path of kundalini, he begins to understand that a number of hatha practices are designed to trigger initial stirring in the energy channels. Where previously the word *hatha* meant to him only a "forcing of the body" as shown in the lexicons, now he suddenly sees it as a process leading to the kundalini by the solar path (of which the *bīja,* or seed sound, is *ha*) and the lunar path (of which the *bīja* is *tha*). To him, then, *nauli* (for instance) becomes a process of awakening the solar plexus and not merely an exercise to keep the body trim.

Of special value in this connection are the *mudrās* (seals) and *bandhas* (locks). The *mudrās* such as *ashvini* and *mahāmudra* appear to be mere physical practices, but they are meant to awaken states of energy channels. The *bandhas* are of two kinds:

a. Those with an apparent physical function, for example, *jālandhara-bandha,* the chin lock. To an uninitiated *sādhaka,* the only purpose of this lock is to hold the breath in during *kumbhaka.* In kundalini yoga, however, the lock controls the upward flow of energy.

b. Those with no apparent physical purpose, initially. For example, the purpose of *mūla-bandha,* the root lock, and the finger locks does not become clear until the energy channels are really activated.

Such hatha yoga practices serve as preparations for the states described under maxim 6: The changes in the subtle body and the energy channels induce changes on the physical plane.

When, by the kind guru's grace, the kundalini begins to ascend, a *sādhaka* leaves the ranks of the slow ones and goes somewhat swifter: as a *madhya* if he is a householder, and as an *adhimātra* if he is a celibate *sanyāsin* (renunciate, monk). In both cases the one-pointed and upward flow (*ekāgratā* and *ūrdhva-gati*) of the kundalini causes certain physiological changes, much as the pattern of the iron filings, in our earlier example, would be altered if the magnetic force changed its directions. Some examples:

a. The body heat, *tapas,* increases.

b. The root lock becomes natural, *sahaja,* and almost permanent, *sthira,* as the prana pulls the forces upward from *mukta-triveṇī* toward *yukta-triveṇī,* from the root center toward the pineal center.

c. The tongue automatically curls back and up toward the palate, thus forming the *khecharī* seal.

d. Not only do the fingers of the hand form the *jñāna-mudra* (the thumb touching the index finger), but the circuit of energy current is so well closed that a pull between the thumb and the finger is felt.

e. An inward turning of the eyes is experienced, often curling the toes upward; this happens at the *gāndhārī* and *hastijihvā* channels.

f. The breath becomes more relaxed and deeper.

g. A general relaxation of limbs takes place in meditation, so that the *sādhaka* might even complain of his arms and hands feeling heavy.

h. The spine straightens itself out because of the prana force.

i. The stomach and the navel area may pull inward, tending toward a natural (*sahaja*) *uḍḍīyāna* lock.

j. The processes of elimination become more efficient, to the point of giving the *sādhaka,* initially, a fear of suffering from diarrhea if his diet is not under control.

This list is by no means exhaustive.

It is with a view to such physiological signs and symptoms of meditative practice that the gurus often tell the disciples, "This will happen by itself." It is then that a *sādhaka* understands the truth of the next maxim: The former (changes in the subtle body) are primary, the latter (changes on the physical plane) auxiliary preparations. In other words, the physical preparations are auxiliary to the primary step in yoga, the awakening of subtler forces.

The path of the *mṛdu* ones is more from the auxiliary toward the primary. In the case of the *madhya* and *adhimātra*, some progress on the inner plane is possible without initially forcing the physical practice. It is especially so in the case of the *adhimātras* who have attained certain interiorization (*antaa-pravṛtti*) in previous incarnations and whom the physical bonds do not impede greatly. Their body cooperates with the inward urge. This does not mean that for the *sādhakas* other than *mṛdus* that physical preparation is unnecessary. The absence of the auxiliary preparations delays progress in the primary ones. The primary then forces the auxiliary. The prior preparation of the auxiliary prevents delay.

The body without spirit is rigid and unconscious (*jada*). Any flexibility in it is due to the forces of *chit*. The rigidity of the body can become a great impediment, for a time at least, when the subtler forces are being awakened. It is better to whittle down the *tamas,* physical inertia of the body, by a constant process of *saṁskāra* purification through a practice of the relevant aspects of hatha yoga, in anticipation of the time when the inner forces will beckon the body to rearrange itself along the newly realized or intensified currents of energy. If the body is too rigid and not ready to cooperate immediately, the progress will be held back until the body is trained appropriately. Some examples can be given here:

a. When the tongue begins to form the *khecharī* seal, it will still fail to block the wastage of *amṛta* (which flows down from *ojas* in deep meditation) if the tongue has not been lengthened sufficiently.

b. The bones and muscles will protest and will interrupt meditation; when the prana is forcing the spine straight, the back muscles will resist.

c. If *uḍḍīyāna* has not been mastered or if the stomach and intestines are not properly cleansed, problems will arise when the prana rising to higher *chakras* will want to pull the *maṇipūra* (the navel center) along. Often, when mind becomes concentrated in a higher center, the prana tries to pull *apāna* (the lower energies) upward; a *sahaja kumbhaka* (natural retention of breath) forms but is impeded if the *uḍḍīyāna* (navel lock) is insufficiently mastered. This can keep a *sādhaka* back for months. It becomes a struggle between the *sattvic* stillness of the mind and the *tamasic* rigidity of the abdominal and stomach muscles.

d. This *sādhaka* (the author) was once advised by the venerable Gurudev to practice *danta-mudra,* clenching the teeth in a certain way during meditation. Like all *sādhakas* who are blessed with the guru's ever-forgiving love and who consequently take freedom to be a little naughty, this *sādhaka* said to himself: Well, what on earth can teeth have to do with meditation? The *danta-mudra* was not practiced. Then came a time when the prana rising up through the straight spine found one loose area to shake up: the hinges of the jaw. The jaw began to move sideways, left and right, during meditation: It stopped only after the *danta-mudra* was perfected. A lesson of obedience to the guru was learnt thus. What was previously a *rahasya* then became real. The inner primary experience forced the auxiliary physical practice. Meanwhile, the progress of prana was kept back, which a prior practice of the physical *mudrā* would have prevented.

The practice of the physical aspects of yoga should be undertaken with a view to preparing the body in anticipation of changes that spiritual progress will (*a*) require, and (*b*) induce or force. The practice, then, should not be ignored, or else problems arising later will slow down the progress in the inner force fields. The practice of hatha yoga should not be overemphasized in isolation from the general spiritual aims. To practice it only for health, beauty, and longevity without any pursuit of deeper truths is to reduce yoga to the level of other physical sciences; it is to ignore the principle that the gross is always an instrument of the sublime. As one progresses, hatha yoga practices at first help and then give way to kundalini yoga. Then an entry into the subtle body is gained.

The path from the gross to the subtle body is more complex than a maze. One cannot be said to have gotten the key to the subtle body unless one has so mastered its use that he can enter it at will. The hatha escorts one to this point and then bids adieu.

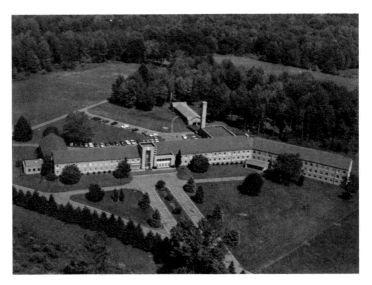

The main building of the national headquarters, Honesdale, Pa.

The Himalayan Institute

The Himalayan International Institute of Yoga Science and Philosophy of the U.S.A. is a nonprofit organization devoted to the scientific and spiritual progress of modern humanity. Founded in 1971 by Sri Swami Rama, the Institute combines Western and Eastern teachings and techniques to develop educational, therapeutic, and research programs for serving people in today's world. The goals of the Institute are to teach meditational techniques for the growth of individuals and their society, to make known the harmonious view of world religions and philosophies, and to undertake scientific research for the benefit of humankind.

This challenging task is met by people of all ages, all walks of life, and all faiths who attend and participate in the Institute courses and seminars. These programs, which are given on a continuing basis, are designed in order that one may discover for oneself how to live more creatively. In the words of Swami Rama, "By being aware of one's own potential and abilities, one can become a perfect citizen, help the nation, and serve humanity."

The Institute has branch centers and affiliates throughout the United States. The 422-acre campus of the national headquarters, located in the Pocono Mountains of northeastern Pennsylvania, serves as the coordination center for all the Institute activities, which include a wide variety of innovative programs in education, research, and therapy, combining Eastern and Western approaches to self-awareness and self-directed change.

SEMINARS, LECTURES, WORKSHOPS, and CLASSES are available throughout the year, providing intensive training and experience in such topics as Superconscious Meditation, hatha yoga, philosophy, psychology, and various aspects of personal growth and holistic health. The *Himalayan News*, a free bimonthly publication, announces the current programs.

The RESIDENTIAL and SELF-TRANSFORMATION PROGRAMS provide training in the basic yoga disciplines—diet, ethical behavior, hatha yoga, and meditation. Students are also given guidance in a philosophy of living in a community environment.

The PROGRAM IN EASTERN STUDIES AND COMPARATIVE PSYCHOLOGY is the first curriculum offered by an educational institution that provides a systematic synthesis of Western empirical sciences with Eastern introspective sciences using both practical and traditional approaches to education. The University of Scranton, by an agreement of affiliation with the Himalayan Institute, is prepared to grant credits for coursework in this program, and upon successful completion of the program awards a Master of Science degree.

The five-day STRESS MANAGEMENT/PHYSICAL FITNESS PROGRAM offers practical and individualized training that can be used to control the stress response. This includes biofeedback, relaxation skills, exercise, diet, breathing techniques, and meditation.

A yearly INTERNATIONAL CONGRESS, sponsored by the Institute, is devoted to the scientific and spiritual progress of modern humanity. Through lectures, workshops, seminars, and practical demonstrations, it provides a forum for professionals and lay people to share their knowledge and research.

The ELEANOR N. DANA RESEARCH LABORATORY is the psychophysiological laboratory of the Institute, specializing in research on breathing, meditation, holistic therapies, and stress and relaxed states. The laboratory is fully equipped for exercise stress testing and psychophysiological measurements, including brain waves, patterns of respiration, heart rate changes, and muscle tension. The staff investigates Eastern teachings through studies based on Western experimental techniques.

Himalayan Institute Publications

Living with the Himalayan Masters	Swami Rama
Lectures on Yoga	Swami Rama
A Practical Guide to Holistic Health	Swami Rama
Choosing a Path	Swami Rama
Inspired Thoughts of Swami Rama	Swami Rama
Freedom from the Bondage of Karma	Swami Rama
Book of Wisdom (Ishopanishad)	Swami Rama
Enlightenment Without God	Swami Rama
Exercise Without Movement	Swami Rama
Life Here and Hereafter	Swami Rama
Marriage, Parenthood, and Enlightenment	Swami Rama
Perennial Psychology of the Bhagavad Gita	Swami Rama
Emotion to Enlightenment	Swami Rama, Swami Ajaya
Science of Breath	Swami Rama, Rudolph Ballentine, M.D., Alan Hymes, M.D.
Yoga and Psychotherapy	Swami Rama, Rudolph Ballentine, M.D., Swami Ajaya
Superconscious Meditation	Usharbudh Arya, D.Litt.
Mantra and Meditation	Usharbudh Arya, D.Litt.
Philosophy of Hatha Yoga	Usharbudh Arya, D.Litt.
Meditation and the Art of Dying	Usharbudh Arya, D.Litt.
God	Usharbudh Arya, D.Litt.
Psychotherapy East and West: A Unifying Paradigm	Swami Ajaya, Ph.D.
Yoga Psychology	Swami Ajaya, Ph.D.
Foundations of Eastern and Western Psychology	Swami Ajaya (ed.)
Psychology East and West	Swami Ajaya (ed.)
Meditational Therapy	Swami Ajaya (ed.)
Diet and Nutrition	Rudolph Ballentine, M.D.
Joints and Glands Exercises	Rudolph Ballentine, M.D. (ed.)
Freedom from Stress	Phil Nuernberger, Ph.D.

Science Studies Yoga	James Funderburk, Ph.D.
Homeopathic Remedies	Drs. Anderson, Buegel, Chernin
Hatha Yoga Manual I	Samskrti and Veda
Hatha Yoga Manual II	Samskrti and Judith Franks
Seven Systems of Indian Philosophy	R. Tigunait, Ph.D.
Swami Rama of the Himalayas	L. K. Misra, Ph.D. (ed.)
Philosophy of Death and Dying	M. V. Kamath
Practical Vedanta of Swami Rama Tirtha	Brandt Dayton (ed.)
The Swami and Sam	Brandt Dayton
Himalayan Mountain Cookery	Martha Ballentine
The Yoga Way Cookbook	Himalayan Institute
Inner Paths	Himalayan Institute
Meditation in Christianity	Himalayan Institute
Art and Science of Meditation	Himalayan Institute
Faces of Meditation	Himalayan Institute
Therapeutic Value of Yoga	Himalayan Institute
Chants from Eternity	Himalayan Institute
Thought for the Day	Himalayan Institute
Spiritual Diary	Himalayan Institute
Blank Books	Himalayan Institute

Write for a free mail order catalog describing all our
publications.